Health
The No-Nonsense Guide
Volume 1

© 2017 Healthful Publications
info.healthful@gmail.com

ALL RIGHTS RESERVED. This book contains material protected under International and Federal Copyright Laws and Treaties. Any unauthorized reprint or use of this material is prohibited. No part of this book may be reproduced or transmitted in any form or by any means, electronic or mechanical, including photocopying, recording, or by any information storage and retrieval system without express written permission from the author / publisher.

This book js not intended as a substitute for the medical advice of physicians. The reader should regularly consult a physician in matters relating to his/her health, particularly with respect to any symptoms that may require diagnosis or medical attention. All readers are advised to seek medical and professional counsel before making any changes to their lifestyle and eating habits.

Table of Contents

TABLE OF CONTENTS..2

INTRODUCTION..4

HOW THE GUT WORKS..7

DIVERTICULOSIS AND DIVERTICULITIS...................12

WHAT IS DIVERTICULITIS?...13
WHAT CAUSES DIVERTICULITIS? 17
SYMPTOMS ASSOCIATED WITH DIVERTICULITIS...............22
DIAGNOSING DIVERTICULITIS.......................................24
HOW TO PREVENT DIVERTICULITIS AND ITS ATTACKS.......27
SURGERIES TO REMOVE DIVERTICULITIS........................33
RECENT ADVANCEMENTS IN SCIENCE 36
CONCLUSION...39

IRRITABLE BOWEL SYNDROME 41

WHAT IS IBS?...42
WHAT CAUSES IBS?...45
SYMPTOMS OF IBS...48
DIAGNOSING IBS 50
YOUR TREATMENT PLAN 52
RECENT ADVANCEMENTS IN SCIENCE 58
CONCLUSION...60

CANDIDA..62

THE NO-NONSENSE GUIDE TO DIGESTIVE DISEASES

BACTERIA AND ITS PURPOSE 63
WHAT IS CANDIDA? 67
WHAT CAUSES CANDIDA OVERGROWTH?......................70
THE SYMPTOMS ASSOCIATED WITH CANDIDA OVERGROWTH 74
DIAGNOSING CANDIDA OVERGROWTH 79
YOUR TREATMENT PLAN 83
RECENT ADVANCEMENTS IN SCIENCE 93
CONCLUSION...96

LEAKY GUT SYNDROME 98

WHAT IS LEAKY GUT SYNDROME?.................................99
WHAT CAUSES LEAKY GUT SYNDROME?......................102
THE SYMPTOMS ASSOCIATED WITH LEAKY GUT SYNDROME 107
DIAGNOSING LEAKY GUT SYNDROME 110
YOUR 4 STEP TREATMENT PLAN 116
RECENT ADVANCEMENTS IN SCIENCE 123
CONCLUSION..128
SOURCES 130

HEALTHFUL PUBLICATIONS

Introduction

"Take all that is given whether wealth, love or language, nothing comes by mistake and with good digestion all can be turned to health" ~ George Herbert

THE NO-NONSENSE GUIDE TO DIGESTIVE DISEASES

When we think of vital organs in the human body what comes to mind? The brain? The heart? The lungs? The gut is an extremely important part of the human physiology that hosts a forgotten organ, gut microflora. Collectively, these organs contribute to the digestion of the food we eat as well as aiding in nutrient absorption that fuels our journey throughout life. The gut microflora is one of many factors that alter how the digestive system functions. Unfortunately millions of people around the globe are suffering from gut malfunctions. This book discusses four disorders in particular; Diverticulosis, Irritable Bowel Syndrome, Candida Overgrowth & Leaky Gut Syndrome.

This book draws from reliable information and removes the unnecessary filler. All quoted sources are from scientific papers, journals, studies or governmental websites. None of the information in this book is sourced from misleading websites or non-scientific sources. If you're interested in understanding the essence of these diseases, how they affect

HEALTHFUL PUBLICATIONS

the human body and the most recent scientific studies explained in everyday understandable terms, you're in the right place.

THE NO-NONSENSE GUIDE TO DIGESTIVE DISEASES

How the Gut Works

"Happiness: a good bank account, a good cook, and a good digestion" ~ Jean-Jacques Rousseau

HEALTHFUL PUBLICATIONS

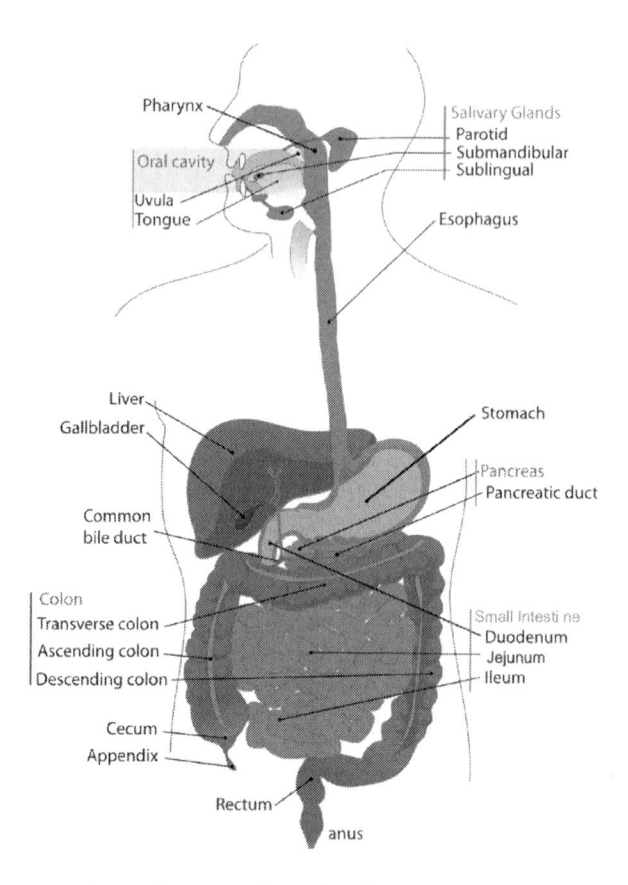

First things first, it is beneficial to gain a wider understanding of how the gut works in its entirety. If you're already well-versed in how the gut operates and strictly want to know about a specific disorder, feel free to skip this

THE NO-NONSENSE GUIDE TO DIGESTIVE DISEASES

part. A refresher is always handy.

The digestive system starts to work from the moment food reaches your mouth and ends when it leaves your body. Food travels through a long tube with many twists and turns, being pushed through a series of processes that allow the body to absorb nutrients and remove waste. This tube is known by names such as the alimentary canal, the gastrointestinal tract (GI tract/GIT), the digestive tract or the gut. The gut starts at the oral cavity (the mouth) and continues into the pharynx, oesophagus, stomach, small intestine and finally the large intestine (which compromises of the cecum, colon, rectum and anal canal).

The process of digestion begins as soon as food enters the mouth. This food is broken into smaller particles by mixing it with salivary enzymes when we chew. This concoction is then passed into the stomach. The stomach introduces new enzymes that are coupled with its highly acidic environment to break food into smaller subunits and is also used as a storage tank, allowing the rest of the gut to finish its processes if the body has consumed a lot of food. The proteins, carbohydrates, fats and other components are broken down into their smaller sub-units such as peptides/amino acids, sugars, and lipids respectively. These smaller sub-units are what the body uses to produce energy for our daily activities and contribute to our maintenance.

These nutrients are then passed into the small intestine which is where the majority of our nutrients are absorbed. Further enzymes from the pancreas combined with bile from the liver are then squeezed through ducts into the small intestine. The small intestine is made up of specialised cells that are adept at latching on to nutrients and absorbing them as food passes through. These nutrients are then transferred into the bloodstream, where they are sent throughout the body for use by various organs. The waste product is then passed into the large intestine which absorbs any remaining nutrients and water before flushing the remaining waste out of the system.

Therefore, the intestines play a central role in the process of digesting and absorbing nutrients and distributing them to the rest of

THE NO-NONSENSE GUIDE TO DIGESTIVE DISEASES

the body. The integrity of the intestinal walls allow the exchange of nutrients between the intestines and the body to be controlled precisely. The intestine is also home to billions of beneficial micro-organisms that help to digest the food we eat. You may have heard of these micro-organisms by their various aliases: microflora or microbiota to name a few. Some bacteria are heavily relied upon to produce enzymes that break down carbohydrates the body cannot.

People suffering with digestive disorders can disrupt their digestive system and upset the balance of the microflora ecosystem. These people are more susceptible to other diseases such as Leaky Gut Syndrome and Candida Overgrowth.

HEALTHFUL PUBLICATIONS

Diverticulosis and Diverticulitis

"The physiologist who succeeds in penetrating deeper and deeper into the digestive canal becomes convinced that it consists of a number of chemical laboratories equipped with various mechanical devices" ~ Ivan Pavlov

THE NO-NONSENSE GUIDE TO DIGESTIVE DISEASES

What is Diverticulitis?

Diverticular disease is simply split into two major stages: Diverticulosis and Diverticulitis. Diverticulosis is a condition characterised by tiny pouches along the large intestine known as diverticula, or diverticulum if only one is present. These tiny pouches are created by consistent strain of passing hard stools. This is why older people are more susceptible to this disease, as the intestines weaken with age[3]. The constant passing of food through the large intestines means that this is quite a common ailment.

A recent scientific review of current diverticular disease classifications has broken this into three stages; Uncomplicated Disease, Chronic Complicated Disease & Acute Complicated Disease. Acute Complicated Disease has 4 sub-classifications, these can be seen below[1]. For the purposes of simplification, this book will discuss diverticular disease in the two major stages as they are common terms that doctors use; Diverticulosis & Diverticulitis.

HEALTHFUL PUBLICATIONS

Uncomplicated Disease

Pain in lower left quadrant, fever, changes in relief pattern.

Chronic Complicated Disease

Impaired passage of stool, recurrent rectal blood loss, incapacitating complaints, high-risk patients, fistula (abnormal connection between two body parts).

Acute Complicated Disease

1. Fever & painful mass
2. Painful obstruction of the intestine
3. Massive rectal blood loss
4. Generalised peritonitis (inflammation of the thin tissue in the inner wall of the abdomen)

    Diverticulitis is what occurs after these bulges become severely irritated and inflamed, turning into pouches. Diverticulitis is the main stage of this disease; luckily, most people experiencing Diverticulosis will not experience Diverticulitis. During Diverticulitis, a number of nasty things can happen to the diverticula. Bacteria can become trapped inside the

THE NO-NONSENSE GUIDE TO DIGESTIVE DISEASES

pouches, abscesses can form in the intestines and stool may get lodged inside a pouch. These symptoms are uncommon. The typical pain caused by Diverticulitis is comparable to indigestion. However, it's vital to make sure a patient with either disorder prevents inflammation and irritation to diverticula. This can mean anything from removing foods from everyday diet or in some cases, a complete lifestyle change. In fact, scientists were able to produce a form of diverticulosis experimentally by feeding rabbits a specific diet[2]. Although reducing the chance of developing Diverticulitis is more than enough of an incentive, most proposed lifestyle changes will grant better health overall.

If you are experiencing Diverticulosis you are not alone; it is estimated that 5% of people have a diverticula by the time they reach 40 years old and 50% of people will have them by the time they are 80 years old[3]. In England during 2010, there were roughly 80,000 hospital admissions alone[4]. Although both men and women are equally likely to suffer from this disease, men under 50 years old are more likely to experience it than women. Interestingly, diverticular disease is often described as a 'western disease' because of the extremely high amount of cases found in Europe and North America and the low amount of cases in African and Asian countries. This is why diet and genes are considered to be the biggest factors in acquiring this disease, often linking it to the lower fibre intake in western countries[4].

What Causes Diverticulitis?

Diverticulitis is an extremely difficult disease to discuss. It's common yet the exact cause isn't entirely understood. The medical community has largely attributed it to genetics and age, two factors that can't be influenced[3]. However, there have been some particularly interesting insights into this field. Below is a list of possible causes for the triggering of this disease.

Genetics

As previously mentioned, western people are more susceptible to developing this disease. Interestingly, people that live in western countries normally develop Diverticulosis in the last third of the colon, while the relatively few patients in Asian countries (such as Japan, Taiwan and Singapore) seem to develop Diverticulosis in the first section of the colon. It's also been noted that the Japanese population living in Hawaii are at a higher risk of Diverticulosis than those living in Japan, but they still develop it in the 'Japanese' location; which is the first part of the colon[5].

Age

Age is commonly linked to Diverticulitis because of the continual weakening of the intestines throughout their use[3]. The figures correlate directly with age; the older you are, the more chance you have of suffering from Diverticulitis. Although the link is very simple to make, it is possible that the actual cause isn't as straightforward as linking one number to another and proclaiming diverticular disease is inevitable.

Straining & Fibre

Since diverticula can be caused by increased pressure when items pass through the intestine, it is entirely possible that people experiencing frequent constipation are prone to Diverticulosis. Constipation is defined by the National Digestive Diseases Information Clearinghouse (NDDIC) of the U.S. to be: "a condition in which an adult has fewer than three bowel movements a week or has bowel movements with stools that are hard, dry, and

THE NO-NONSENSE GUIDE TO DIGESTIVE DISEASES

small, making them painful or difficult to pass"[6].

We normally associate constipation with the inability to have bowel movements. Using the definition above, it is entirely possible to have constipation with frequent bowel movements but with harder than normal stools. Diets high in fibre help to soften stools. Scientists were able to replicate Diverticulosis by feeding rabbits a refined diet of "white bread, butter, sugar, milk and vitamin supplements" further proving that low fibre is a major cause[2]. However, be careful of excessive grain consumption. Grains and omega-6 fatty acids are known to irritate gut lining, so a diet rich in these foods will be more inclined to exacerbate symptoms[7].

Inflammation

Inflammation to the intestinal wall can cause Diverticulosis and aggravate diverticula, even rupturing it. Although it is widely accepted that moderate inflammation is dangerous to those suffering with Diverticulosis, chronic low-grade inflammation can also cause Diverticulosis. Approximately 75% of a 930-patient study that undertook surgery for diverticular disease showed signs of chronic inflammation around the diverticula[8].

What causes inflammation of the intestinal wall? Other gut disorders such as IBS, Candida Overgrowth and Leaky Gut Syndrome can contribute to an irritated gut lining. Non-steroidal anti-inflammatory drugs (NSAIDs), such as ibuprofen are also known to cause complications. High levels of stress have been well documented to cause a variety of negative affects to the intestines, one of which is inflammation[9].

Intestinal Bacteria

As bacteria can enter diverticula pouches and cause infection, by understanding how to reduce the chances of this happening and defining the culprits, you can better equip yourself.

The gut is home to trillions of bacteria. Our gut is inhabited by a collective group of good and bad bacteria, otherwise known as our gut flora or microbiota/microbiome. Our gut microbiome contributes tremendously to our

THE NO-NONSENSE GUIDE TO DIGESTIVE DISEASES

everyday lives, unbeknownst to many. They protect us from organisms that attack our intestines[10,11]; they assist in the absorption of nutrients and energy from the food we eat[12,13] (even foods that our body is unable to digest alone); and they help our immune system work at full capacity[14]. In fact, tests that study the effect of probiotic bacteria and antibiotic drugs suggest that the microbiome regulates anxiety, mood, cognition and pain[15]. A bacterial overgrowth observed in patients with Diverticulosis or an unbalanced bacterial ecosystem, has been linked to intestinal inflammation.

If you have previously taken a large dose of antibiotics it is important to take the necessary steps to increase the amounts of good bacteria and achieve symbiosis.

HEALTHFUL PUBLICATIONS

Symptoms Associated with Diverticulitis

There are varying degrees of symptoms in patients with diverticular disease. A particularly frequent symptom is a re-occurring pain in the stomach, often in the lower left side of the abdomen for western people or right side for Asian people. This pain can worsen during or shortly after a meal. Passing stools may relieve the pain. Other symptoms include[3]:

- Constipation, diarrhoea or periods of constipation followed by diarrhoea
- Bloating
- Bleeding from the rectum

Once Diverticulosis has advanced into its more severe stage of Diverticulitis, the pain becomes noticeably more severe and constant. The pain starts below the belly button and moves to the usual area; the lower left side of the abdomen for Western people or right side for Asian people. Other symptoms include:

THE NO-NONSENSE GUIDE TO DIGESTIVE DISEASES

- High temperatures of and exceeding 38 degrees Celsius or 100 degrees Fahrenheit
- Feeling or being sick
- Constipation
- Bleeding from the rectum
- Frequent urination
- Difficulty or pain while urinating

HEALTHFUL PUBLICATIONS

Diagnosing Diverticulitis

Diverticular disease is a tricky condition to diagnose from symptoms alone. However, if anyone experiences the symptoms previously mentioned, it is important to see a doctor immediately.

It is difficult to successfully diagnose Diverticulitis at first glance as it shares similar symptoms with other digestive disorders. Doctors are likely to run a series of tests to rule out easily identifiable diseases. A blood test will likely be recommended to rule out coeliac disease. Urine tests will allow signs of infection to be checked. Pregnancy tests may be suggested to women of childbearing age to negate pregnancy as the cause of abdominal pain. Liver function tests negate the possibility of abdominal pain caused by conditions such as alcohol-related liver disease. A stool test may be taken from those that are experiencing diarrhoea in order to rule out further infections.

There are a variety of tests a doctor can run if he/she suspects that the symptoms match

THE NO-NONSENSE GUIDE TO DIGESTIVE DISEASES

with digestive disorders such as Diverticulosis[3].

Colonoscopy

When symptoms align with Diverticulosis or Diverticulitis a doctor may advise a colonoscopy. A colonoscopy is the easiest way of looking directly inside the large intestine to check for any bulges or pouches that look like diverticula. During a colonoscopy, a colonoscope is placed into the rectum and further into the colon that houses the pain. A colonoscope is a thin tube that has a camera attached to the end. Laxatives are prescribed beforehand to empty the bowels and allow for an easier diagnosis. Although this sounds extremely uncomfortable, the procedure isn't normally painful. However, the patient may be given a sedative or painkilling medication beforehand so as to reduce any feelings of discomfort.

Barium enema X-ray

Barium is a special liquid, it is used to cover the colon so as to make it easier to see in X-rays. Barium is special as it coats the inside of organs, allowing hidden parts of organs such as the colon to be displayed. This allows a doctor to investigate how the colon looks and if there are any visible bulges or pouches. Firstly, a laxative will be provided to clear out the colon. A tube will then be inserted into the rectum, squirting the barium into the tube and up through the rectum. A few X-rays will then be taken. Do not worry if stool appears white or discoloured for a few days afterwards, this is just the barium safely leaving your body.

CT scans

Patients that have had a blood test show an unusually high number of white blood cells (which indicates infection) or have a history of diverticular disease may cause a doctor to assume diverticular disease. However, a CT scan may be used to rule out other conditions such as gallstones or a hernia. CT or computerised tomography scans take a series of X-rays which are displayed on a computer to build a 3-D image. CT scans are beneficial as they allow large areas to be visualised, which is particularly useful when infections have spread. This may be the case in complications such as abscesses.

THE NO-NONSENSE GUIDE TO
DIGESTIVE DISEASES

How to Prevent Diverticulitis and its Attacks

Unfortunately, there is no known cure for Diverticulosis or Diverticulitis. However, there are some preventative measures that can be taken to reduce the chance of Diverticular based attacks from happening. Since over 50% of people aged 80 and older are likely to suffer from Diverticulosis, the following actions should be considered as safety precautions. It's better to be safe than sorry.

Fibre & Diet

A low-fibre diet is widely considered to be the triggering factor behind Diverticulosis. As previously explained, it is thought that consistent hard stools or straining during bowel movements contribute to forming diverticula. If a diet consists of low amounts of fibre, then stools will become harder and more difficult to pass. Therefore, it is recommended to increase the amount of fibre intake, either through diet or supplements[16]. 20 to 38 grams of fibre is recommended each day to prevent Diverticulosis[16].

Foods rich in fibre include: fresh fruits, vegetables, beans, lentils etc. Be wary of consuming an excess of grains however, as mentioned in the previous chapter there is evidence to suggest that grains can worsen symptoms. If you are struggling to eat enough fibre, another tactic is to include foods of liquid consistency such as soups or vegetable based juices to soften the consistency of stools. Strong evidence shows that insoluble fibre found in fruits and vegetables decrease risk of diverticular disease more effectively than their soluble counterpart. There is also some evidence indicating that the combination of high red meat consumption coupled with low fibre particularly increases the risk of diverticular disease[17]. As of now, alcohol, caffeine and smoking do not appear to influence diverticular disease, but they are known to irritate the digestive system[18].

THE NO-NONSENSE GUIDE TO DIGESTIVE DISEASES

Eliminate straining

Straining causes undue pressure on the intestines. It's important to be mindful during bowel movements and eliminate as much straining as possible. Even a small amount of straining over a long period of time is enough to weaken the intestines. A high fibre diet reduces the need to strain.

Restore intestinal flora

As mentioned previously, an unbalanced gut flora (dysbiosis) may also contribute to Diverticulitis. The gut flora assist the body in a variety of different manners; including improving mood and the immune system. By restoring balance in the intestinal flora, it'll allow the digestive function to operate normally as well as improve overall health. This is particularly important after the digestion of strong antibiotics as they kill both good and bad bacteria in a non-selective manner. To remedy this, take probiotics and prebiotics. Probiotics are a collection of live bacteria that can be found in yogurt and other dairy products, while prebiotics are a specialised plant fibre that good bacteria consume to fuel themselves[19].

Reducing intestinal inflammation

The best way to reduce both intestinal inflammation and the chances of causing diverticula is by careful diet monitoring. Foods such as grains and omega-6 fatty acids are known to cause inflammation and must be avoided at all costs. Similarly, NSAIDs such as ibuprofen must also be avoided[20,21]. Instead, consume omega-9 fatty acids, found in foods such as olives and avocados, omega-3 fatty acids in fish, garlic, herbs such as basil, oregano, parsley and turmeric, and green tea. All of these foods are found to reduce inflammation as well as overall health.

Eliminate stress

Stress continuously weakens the body, especially the gut[22]. It's easy to acknowledge when you're stressed but it's harder to act on it. Most people take stress as a necessity, whether it's caused by work, family or everyday life. There are simple ways to control and reduce stress in a world that is uncontrollable. Activities such as meditation, yoga and Tai Chi

THE NO-NONSENSE GUIDE TO DIGESTIVE DISEASES

are very popular in today's society. Even 10 minutes of meditation a day can reduce stress, increase concentration and act as a pick-me-up when needed most. Regular participation of these activities grants control over stress and emotions that are otherwise hard to manage.

Supplements

Preventing Diverticulitis can require a lifestyle change and a lot of effort. There are a vast amount of supplements that allow us to meet certain requirements that may be hard to manage. Below is a list of supplements and the areas they benefit:

Fibre:

- Psyllium Husk Capsules
- Fruit Cubes
- Fibre Capsules
- Partially Hydrolysed Guar Gum

Intestinal Flora:

- Acidophilus
- Probiotics that include Escherichia Coli strain Nissle 1917 or Probiotics in general

HEALTHFUL PUBLICATIONS

- Prebiotics

Inflammation:

- Omega 3s or Fish Oil Capsules
- Vitamin C Tablets
- Vitamin E Tablets
- Bioflavanoids found in things such as Grape Seed Extract or Garlic Capsules. They are also found in onions and apples
- Garlic capsules
- Co-enzyme Q10
- Milk Thistle to reduce inflammation in the liver if needed

THE NO-NONSENSE GUIDE TO DIGESTIVE DISEASES

Surgeries to Remove Diverticulitis

Historically, surgeries were offered to those that had suffered from two or more Diverticulitis attacks as a provision to protect against future attacks and complications. This has changed recently and now the general consensus is that the costs of surgery outweigh the benefits; an estimated 1 in 100 suffer from complications after surgery[3]. There are exceptions to this rule. Reoccurring complications or consistent suffering from a young age may merit surgery to prolong suffering, since the longer someone lives with this disease the higher the chances of complications. There are two main types of surgery associated with Diverticulitis.

Stoma Surgery

In situations where the large intestine is severely damaged, it is recommended that the intestine heal for a minimum of nine weeks so as to fully recover. This is where stoma surgery

HEALTHFUL PUBLICATIONS

is used. A stoma is a small hole in the abdomen that allows waste to pass out into a man-made pouch, bypassing the intestine altogether. There are two types of stoma surgeries.

Ileostomy – The stoma is situated in the stomach. The large intestine is isolated from the small intestine and sealed, allowing adequate time to heal. The small intestine is diverted and joined to the stoma.

Colostomy – Instead of isolating the large intestine, only a small section is isolated. The rest of the large intestine is joined to the stoma in the lower abdomen.

Colectomy

This method involves removing the troublesome part of the large intestine. This may be performed in two ways; an open colectomy or a laparoscopic colectomy. An open colectomy involves the removal of a section of the large intestine through a large incision in the abdomen, while the laparoscopic colectomy is a type of keyhole surgery.

Surgery is normally successful with an

THE NO-NONSENSE GUIDE TO DIGESTIVE DISEASES

estimated 1 in 12 people having a recurrence of symptoms afterwards[3].

HEALTHFUL PUBLICATIONS

Recent Advancements in Science

Science progresses on a daily basis, so much so that it is hard for general practitioners to keep up-to-date. It's important to note that this does not always mean new information is superior. In fact, studies that have plenty of counter-arguments or are used as a basis for further investigation are the most reliable. Although, it never hurts to stay one step ahead. This section summarises interesting advancements that have occurred in the last few years.

Diagnosis

Discussions of correctly diagnosing diverticular disease are common in recent literature. The first topic relates to differentiating IBS from diverticular disease[23]. This counter-study was originally conducted as a way to investigate claims that people suffering from acute diverticulitis are susceptible to IBS going forwards[24]. This is particularly interesting as the both diseases share common symptoms, which

THE NO-NONSENSE GUIDE TO DIGESTIVE DISEASES

is why it's important that medical practitioners are able to distinguish between the two. The study concludes that 12.8% of acute diverticulitis patients contacted continued to have diverticular related symptoms, which the previous study claimed were IBS related.

A study of 72 patients between 2012 and 2013 set out to discover the single most characterising symptom of uncomplicated diverticular disease[25]. Interestingly, this study also made the distinction between IBS and diverticular disease; stating that by definition, IBS is a disease with no structural or organic lesions. The study concluded that "moderate to severe and prolonged left lower-abdominal pain" is the best identifier of diverticular disease.

Treatments

There is not much information on how probiotics affect diverticular disease but an investigation in 2016 aimed to kick-start it[26]. Unfortunately this study didn't lead to significant evidence swaying either way, but this is an interesting direction to look at in the future.

HEALTHFUL PUBLICATIONS

11%-38% of people that receive endoscopic treatment for diverticular bleeding are re-admitted into the hospital within 30 days[27]. This next study investigated how high-dose barium impaction, barium that is retained after a barium enema x-ray may actually help to lower the risk of recurrent bleeding[28]. Although the outcome of this study was successful, it requires many more studies with much larger sample sizes to be credible.

Finally, and the most interesting evolution. There has been recent development in the technology used to surgically intervene with those from suffering particularly bad diverticular lesions[29]. A special 'over-the-scope clip' can be attached to endoscopes, allowing the surgeon to enter the intestines and insert a clip, closing the lesion, in one minimally invasive procedure.

THE NO-NONSENSE GUIDE TO DIGESTIVE DISEASES

Conclusion

If you or someone close to you is suffering from diverticulosis or diverticulitis attacks it can be emotionally and physically damaging. However, you are not alone. Although we currently do not know the exact reason behind the occurrence of diverticulosis; lack of fibre, consistent straining or constipation seem to be a reoccurring trigger. It is interesting that western people are much more susceptible to these conditions. This is often attributed to differences in genetics and diet.

The amount of people that will develop diverticulosis in their lifetimes is astonishing. Although this disease is currently incurable there are many alternative methods that can reduce the suffering and prevent diverticulosis from turning into diverticulitis. Increasing fibre intake, consuming foods with anti-inflammatory properties such as onions or apples, restoring intestinal flora with probiotics and reducing stress by taking up stress management activities such as meditation or yoga can ease the symptoms of diverticular disease.

As digestive disorders are becoming more frequent so is the attention the medical community provides. Patients are urged to take their health seriously, adopt lifestyle changes and focus on eating habits so as to prevent diverticulitis attacks. By taking small but consistent dietary changes, diverticulitis may be prevented and the discomfort from diverticulosis should be comparable to that of mild indigestion. As time goes on, we will uncover more of the root causes and solutions to this problem. In the meantime there are actionable steps that will grant a healthier, happier life.

THE NO-NONSENSE GUIDE TO DIGESTIVE DISEASES

Irritable Bowel Syndrome

"When I prayed for success, I forgot to ask for sound sleep and good digestion" ~ **Mason Cooley**

HEALTHFUL PUBLICATIONS

What is IBS?

IBS is a functional gastrointestinal disorder, which means that the function of the gut changes but not its physical shape. IBS is tricky to understand as there's no concrete evidence indicating what causes the gut to act so differently. This disorder has had various names in the past; such as colitis, spastic colon, mucous colitis, nervous colon and spastic bowel. It is hard to believe that doctors used to think that IBS was 'all in the head' with no physical triggers[30]. More and more research is proving that IBS is indeed a physical and mental disorder that affects people's lives. In fact, Norwegian medical researchers have taken the first image of an irritable bowel in action and the results are astonishing: http://sciencenordic.com/first-image-irritable-bowel. This is why the name has been altered to better represent the mental and physical causes of this disorder, removing the aspect of hypochondria surrounding previous diagnoses[31].

IBS is not a traditional disorder in which

THE NO-NONSENSE GUIDE TO DIGESTIVE DISEASES

something specific can be diagnosed; it is a cluster of abnormal gut reactions that happen frequently and consistently. Specific types of IBS can be identified to better understand individual treatments; the subcategories are as follows[32]:

IBS with constipation (IBS-C)

- Hard stools more than 25% of the time
- Loose stools less than 25% of the time

IBS with diarrhoea (IBS-D)

- Hard stools less than 25% of the time
- Loose stools more than 25% of the time

IBS-mixed (IBS-M)

- Hard stools more than 25% of the time
- Loose stools more than 25% of the time

IBS-unclassified (IBS-U)

- Hard stools less than 25% of the time
- Loose stools less than 25% of the time

HEALTHFUL PUBLICATIONS

A healthy digestive tract is allows the intestines to contract and expand in a way that lets food pass through in a timely manner. This is thought to change in those that suffer from IBS. A sufferer of IBS-D is thought to pass food through the intestines too quickly and a sufferer of IBS-C passes food too slowly. Interestingly a Chinese study of 754 patients found that 66.3% had IBS-D, 14.7% had IBS-C, 4.2% had IBS-M and 14.8% had IBS-U[33]. The next section discusses what scientific studies have unravelled about the causes of IBS.

THE NO-NONSENSE GUIDE TO DIGESTIVE DISEASES

What Causes IBS?

There is no known cause of IBS but there are a few theories. These range from previous intestinal infections to diets that rely heavily upon certain food groups. Although these theories are promising, there isn't enough scientific research to back up these claims so their direct link to IBS is unknown[34].

Gut Brain Axis

The 'gut-brain axis' allows communication between the gut and brain, both of which assist the body in various ways. If your body is used to eating at a certain time but today has been too hectic to scoff down your sandwich, it will inform the brain of hunger. It can, however, be influenced by other stimuli; for example, when nervous or stressed before an exam, interview or presentation, it may inform the brain that you need the toilet[35].

It's believed that people with IBS may have extremely sensitive digestive nerve signals. This could explain the abnormality in intestinal rhythm and urgencies to use the toilet. It is also interesting to note that indigestion may become much more intense in those with sensitive nerve signals[34].

Common Misconceptions

A study in 2007 aimed at discovering what the general public assume about IBS provided thought-provoking results. It investigated what people already know about IBS and which areas these people would like know more about. It discovered that a large number of people believed certain misconceptions that were either not proven to be true or downright incorrect; 52% believed that IBS is caused by a lack of digestive enzymes, 47.9% believed it worsens with age, 43% believed it can develop into colitis, 42.8% believed it is a form of colitis, 37.7% believed it can develop into malnutrition and 21.4% believed it can develop into cancer[36].

Triggers

Although the exact cause is unknown, common IBS triggers have been identified. In a 2005 study, 64% of individuals with IBS believed it was triggered by a specific food or drink and

THE NO-NONSENSE GUIDE TO DIGESTIVE DISEASES

30% believed it was due to stress[37]. A study in 2008 of 62 sufferers that underwent a low FODMAP diet showed that 74% of those patients obtained and sustained improvement in all of their gut symptoms. Highly fermentable, poorly absorbed short-chain carbohydrates (otherwise known as FODMAPs) can cause problems with digestion. FODMAP stands for **F**ermentable **O**ligo-saccharides, **D**i-saccharides, **M**ono-saccharides, **A**nd **P**olyols. Other foods that are known to exacerbate this problem are also excluded in this diet, such as Fructose, Lactose, Fructans and Galacto-Oligosaccharides[38]. The list of foods that reside under these categories are extensive and are listed in a later section. However, common triggers include lactose (milk), alcohol, caffeine, onions, garlic, gluten and wheat.

HEALTHFUL PUBLICATIONS

Symptoms of IBS

There are a variety of symptoms associated with IBS; some are a direct cause of digestive issues and others are triggered indirectly. The main symptoms include**Error! Bookmark not defined.**:

- Diarrhoea, constipation, or alternating between them

- Flatulence

- Bloating

- Abdominal pain

- Urgency to use the toilet

- A feeling of not fully emptying bowels after using the toilet

- Passing mucus from your rectum

Other symptoms can be brought on as an addition to the main symptoms but are not apparent in all cases of IBS. These are:

- Lethargy

- Nausea

THE NO-NONSENSE GUIDE TO DIGESTIVE DISEASES

- Backache
- Bladder problems
- Pain during sex
- Incontinence

• Depression & Anxiety - these may be brought on by the impact of IBS on everyday life as well as the disruption to the gut-brain axis.

HEALTHFUL PUBLICATIONS

Diagnosing IBS

Since IBS doesn't change the structural integrity of the digestive system, no physical examination can be done to diagnose it[32]. This is why it's important to vividly explain symptoms to a doctor, no matter how embarrassing. If you've had consistent; bloating, abdominal pain, diarrhoea and/or constipation in a six-month period, your doctor is likely to consider you for IBS. They should then ask additional questions to find out if symptoms get worse after eating and if using the toilet relieves them.

The symptoms of many digestive problems are very similar, meaning you may be asked to undertake various tests to make sure you don't suffer from serious digestive issues such as celiac disease. You may be asked to undertake a blood test, urine and/or stool sample. It is even possible to be put forward for a colonoscopy if the symptoms you exhibit are closely related to the symptoms of bowel or ovarian cancer[32]. That is why it is essential to visit a doctor instead of self-diagnosing.

THE NO-NONSENSE GUIDE TO DIGESTIVE DISEASES

HEALTHFUL PUBLICATIONS

Your Treatment Plan

There is no cure for IBS but do not fear, it is possible to reduce the symptoms to such a degree that IBS barely affects your everyday life. This is why it's important to monitor the specific set of triggers that set off these symptoms and carefully avoid them.

Mental Health & Stress

The mind and digestive system work hand-in-hand thanks to the brain-gut axis. Unfortunately, this means that problems can be compounded. For example, if you are constantly aware of digestive issues you're likely to create stress, which in turn increases digestive issues.

Stress continuously weakens the body, especially the gut[22]. It's easy to acknowledge when you're stressed but it's harder to act on it. Most people take stress as a necessity, whether it's caused by work, family or everyday life. There are simple ways to control and reduce stress in a world that is uncontrollable.

THE NO-NONSENSE GUIDE TO DIGESTIVE DISEASES

Activities such as meditation, yoga and Tai Chi are very popular in today's society. Even 10 minutes of meditation a day can reduce stress, increase concentration and act as a pick-me-up when needed most. Regular participation of these activities grants control over stress and emotions that are otherwise hard to manage.

IBS can cause depression and depression-like symptoms[39]. Not only do these mental health issues limit quality of life; they also make it harder to follow a strict recovery plan. This is why both issues should be tackled together. It's important to see a doctor or psychologist to undertake a complete and thorough understanding as the link between depression and IBS isn't straightforward and has much to do with the individual's beliefs and thoughts towards the matter[40].

FODMAP

The information in this section has been sourced from the research adapted by Guy's and St Thomas' NHS Foundation Trust and King's College London FODMAP publications (Parlett, 2014[41]). The information in these

HEALTHFUL PUBLICATIONS

booklets were originally developed in Australia at Monash University in Melbourne. If you would like to purchase these booklets, which I highly recommend, go to www.kcl.ac.uk/fodmaps or ask your dietician. This information is correct as of time of publication.

As mentioned previously, FODMAP stands for **F**ermentable, **O**ligo-saccharides (fructans & galacto-oligosaccharides), **D**i-saccharides (lactose), **M**ono-saccharides (fructose), **A**nd **P**olyols (sugar alcohols). These FODMAPs are certain strains of carbohydrates that are not absorbed in the small intestine and move directly to the large intestine. The bacteria in the large intestine then ferment FODMAPs, which can cause wind, bloating and pain. Osmosis can occur, increasing/decreasing the amount of water in the large intestines, causing diarrhoea or constipation. Reducing these types of carbohydrates can improve symptoms in as short a period as two weeks.

Foods to Avoid

Galacto-oligosaccharides (GOS) are poorly absorbed carbohydrates in most people, which

THE NO-NONSENSE GUIDE TO DIGESTIVE DISEASES

we can't break down. These are found in pulses, legumes, beans and various vegetables. **Particular foods to avoid** include: artichoke, baked beans, lima beans, red beans, chickpeas, lentils and soy beverages. **Foods that shouldn't be eaten in large quantities** include: black-eyed beans, broad beans, butter beans, kidney beans, beetroot, broccoli, fennel, lettuce, onion and peas.

Fructans are also poorly absorbed. This includes the infamous wheat and rye as well as various fruit and vegetables. **Particular foods to avoid** include: artichoke, asparagus, barley, camas bulb, chicory root, dandelion leaves, garlic, leek, all forms of onion and yacon. **Foods that shouldn't be eaten in large quantities** include: banana, beetroot, brussel sprouts, cantaloupe melon, grapefruit, longon, honeydew melon, nectarine, peach, persimmon, rambutan, spinach, watermelon and zucchini.

Lactose may be poorly absorbed, but it isn't always the case. Speak to your doctor or dietician in regards to restricting lactose. Lactose is found in milk and yoghurts.

Fructose may also be poorly absorbed, but this too isn't always the case. Speak to your doctor or dietician in regards to restricting fructose. Fructose is found in various fruits, fruit juices (over 100ml) and honey. It is recommended to only eat one portion of fruit at a time. However, glucose allows fructose to be absorbed more easily, so foods high in both may create few symptoms. **Particular foods to avoid** include: apple, boysenberry, fig, mango, sugar snap peas, fruit juice concentrate in sweets, agave nectar, tropical juices and fructose sweeteners such as; fructose syrup, glucose-fructose syrup, fructose-glucose syrup, high fructose corn syrup and high fructose corn syrup solids. **Foods that can only be eaten in small quantities** include; one banana, a slice of pineapple or honeydew melon, a small bowl of fruit salad or strawberries, 10 grapes, 1-2 clementines, mandarins or kiwifruit, one tablespoon dried fruit e.g. raisins, half a glass of suitable fruit juice (100ml), or one tomato.

Polyols are sugar alcohols. Sorbitol, xylitol and mannitol are the most common. **Particular foods to avoid** include: snow peas, apples, apricots, blackberries, nectarines,

THE NO-NONSENSE GUIDE TO DIGESTIVE DISEASES

mushrooms, peach, pears, plum, watermelon, cherries and large quantities of beer. **Foods that shouldn't be eaten in large quantities** include: avocado, cauliflower, celery, lychee, grapes and sweet potato.

By sticking to a rigorous diet that excludes problematic foods for 8 weeks, symptoms should be dramatically reduced. It is then advised to consult your dietician to create a food plan, reintroducing certain foods. Once again, this data is only for informative purposes. Please consult a doctor or dietician before making any lifestyle changes.

HEALTHFUL PUBLICATIONS

Recent Advancements in Science

Science progresses on a daily basis, so much so that it is hard for general practitioners to keep up-to-date. It's important to note that this does not always mean new information is superior. In fact, studies that have plenty of counter-arguments or are used as a basis for further investigation are the most reliable. Although, it never hurts to stay one step ahead. This section summarises interesting advancements that have occurred in the last few years.

Causation

A study in early 2015 observed that microbial alterations could be a leading cause of IBS. However, this requires much more research as diet takes a large role in manipulating the microbiota, which was not thoroughly investigated in this study[42]. Similarly, a study in the US found that patients prior to gastroenteritis (bacteria or infection that causes vomiting and diarrhoea) had a similar microbial reaction to those with IBS, suggesting people that suffer from an intestinal illness may be predisposed towards IBS[43].

Treatment

Unfortunately there isn't an abundance of new information on solutions to this problem. A meta-analysis of 21 studies demonstrated that focusing on a singular probiotic at a low dosage appeared to improve the overall symptoms and quality of life of patients[44]. This seems to be very promising. It is likely that more studies on specific strains, doses and types of probiotics will be investigated thoroughly in the future.

Lastly, a review of published clinical studies of the FODMAP diet. The review is extremely positive, proving that a low FODMAP diet is the most promising method of reducing IBS like systems and living a normal, happy life[45].

Conclusion

If you or someone close to you is suffering from IBS it can be emotionally and physically damaging. Although it isn't currently possible to reverse this problem and go back to the same routine enjoyed before, there are lifestyle choices that can minimise symptoms, resulting in a life similar to before IBS became an issue. It is extremely important to understand both how bodies react and what's causing IBS. This is why professional diagnosis is vital. Patients with IBS-D, IBS-C, IBS-M and IBS-U all vary in terms of specific symptoms, triggers and treatments.

Addressing both mental and dietary components of the IBS treatment plan will not only counteract the negative effects of IBS but also contribute to a much healthier future. By following a FODMAP diet or any other program aimed at finding the culprits of IBS issues - as directed by a dietician or doctor - as well as seeking mental health support if needed, the triggers of IBS effectively become non-existent. It is also comforting to know that IBS doesn't cause any lasting damage to the physiology of the digestive system.

HEALTHFUL PUBLICATIONS

Candida

"Give me good digestion, Lord, And also something to digest; but where and how that something comes I leave to Thee, who knoweth best" ~ Mary Webb

THE NO-NONSENSE GUIDE TO DIGESTIVE DISEASES

Bacteria and its Purpose

Just a forewarning. This section is reference heavy to ensure the highest level of scientific accuracy. The intention has been to write this section so that everybody can understand it, however there are certain words, phrases and meanings that may be difficult to comprehend. Furthermore, if you're just interested in Candida and aren't interested in how bacteria affects our lives, feel free to skip this chapter.

Our gut is inhabited by a collective group of good and bad bacteria, otherwise known as gut flora or microbiota/microbiome. Our gut microbiome contributes tremendously to our everyday lives, unbeknownst to many. They protect us from organisms that attack our intestines[10,11], they assist in the absorption of nutrients and energy from the food we eat[12,13] (even foods that our body is unable to digest alone) and they help our immune system work at full capacity[14]. In fact, tests that study the effect of probiotic bacteria and antibiotic drugs suggest that the microbiome regulates anxiety, mood, cognition and pain[15]. It is entirely possible that currently 'untreatable' conditions may be caused by activities occurring within our gut that we do not yet understand. What do we know about the microbiota so far?

Currently, there is very little research that studies the effects of certain strains of bacteria in our gut, but that isn't entirely the medical communities fault. There are literally trillions of microbes that inhabit the human intestine, interacting with each other in a complex ecosystem and fulfilling purposes that aren't easy to pinpoint[46].

However, breakthroughs – whether widely accepted or controversial - are being made every day. Soya beans cancer fighting properties have been highly debated, there have been claims that they cause cancer, others claim they fight it[47]. Asian communities have benefitted from their soya rich diets with lower chances of osteoporosis, prostate cancer and cardiovascular disease. All of these benefits have been caused by (s)-equol produced by bacterial enzymes[48]. Japanese, Korean or Chinese people are 25-30% more likely to

THE NO-NONSENSE GUIDE TO DIGESTIVE DISEASES

produce these results than their Western counter-parts, meaning these benefits may only help those with intestines rich in these specific bacterial strains[48].

Although there are certain bacterial species that are known to reside in healthy people, different factors contribute to varied levels of bacteria diversity such as; age and location**Error! Bookmark not defined.**[49]. However, there is one easy to digest, so to speak, general rule that sustains good health; a diverse range of bacteria in the gut is a healthy gut[46].

If a diverse range of bacteria is so important, are we able to influence and control our microbiota in an attempt to improve our overall health? The good news is that it's possible. If an individual changes their diet so as to; reduce their carbohydrate or fat intake for a year, intake high amounts of fat and low fibre, or low amounts of fat and high fibre for 10 days it can make substantial changes in the gut microbiome[46]. Although these changes can occur in a small timespan, a constant routine is necessary to keep particular species healthy in the long-run.

If it's possible to influence our health by introducing good bacteria into our body, then it is entirely possible to negatively impact our health by directly or indirectly harming good bacteria and promoting the rise of bad bacteria.

THE NO-NONSENSE GUIDE TO DIGESTIVE DISEASES

What is Candida?

Candida is a family of fungal organisms that reside in the mouth and intestines in very small quantities. Most species of these fungal organisms are naturally harmless to human health, some even assist with digestive function. These helpful species boost the absorption of nutrients from within the digestive tract. Candida is in fact very important for the overall health and wellbeing of human beings.

The overproduction of these fungal organisms can be extremely dangerous. It is the most common cause for yeast infections worldwide[50]. Candida Albicans (or c. albicans) is a common species that resides within the digestive tract and skin. It is also the main culprit for causing bloodstream infections, known as Candidiasis (or Candidemia).

As previously mentioned in the explanation of the digestive system, the bacterial ecosystem helps support many bodily functions such as nutrient absorption and allowing the immune system to work at full capacity. If this delicate ecosystem is disrupted (known as dysbiosis), it can have a variety of negative effects on the body. A collectively large group of Candida can even break down the wall of the intestine and penetrate into the bloodstream. Once achieved, the fungus is able to release toxic by-products into the internal system of the body, thereby giving rise to a disease condition generally known as Candidiasis. Once Candida has entered the bloodstream it is able to travel to other parts of the body. The specific regions of the body, which this disease can affect, include the skin, genitals, throat, mouth and even the blood. Different names are used to specify each of these types of Candidiasis:

• Candidiasis that affects the mouth or throat is known as oral Candidiasis, oropharyngeal Candidiasis, or thrush.

• Candidiasis that affects the genital region is known as a yeast infection or a vulvovaginal yeast infection (in females).

• Invasive Candidiasis or Candidemia is the

name given to the infection that affects the bloodstream.

This opportunistic yeast infection has been officially documented. Varied levels of infection have been recognized, ranging from minor to life threatening systematic diseases that predominantly affect debilitated patients[51]. Candida is no minor issue. It is vital to be able to be aware of the symptoms associated with an overgrowth so that anyone suffering with this condition can seek proper diagnosis. It is also important to self-educate on various ways that allow a Candida overgrowth to occur.

HEALTHFUL PUBLICATIONS

What Causes Candida Overgrowth?

The first step in accurately diagnosing Candida overgrowth is to identify if an individual has followed actions that make them more susceptible to this disease. As Candida is an opportunistic yeasts, there are a few triggers that can allow such an outbreak to happen.

Overconsumption of refined sugars and carbohydrates: Yeast feed off of sugars such as glucose or fructose, which are common place in store-bought products. Carbohydrates are broken down into glucose to help fuel the body. It is no surprise that diets rich in carbohydrates and sugars promote a high Candida population. There are many foods that are extremely healthy for us but are unfortunately packed with natural sugars, an examples of such foods are; bananas, honey, cherries, mangoes and dried fruit etc. Although healthy, moderation is key. Overconsumption of these foods may give Candida enough fuel to kick start its rise to overgrowth.

THE NO-NONSENSE GUIDE TO DIGESTIVE DISEASES

Taking antibiotics: The fact that antibiotic drugs are exceptional at killing both bad and good bacteria is not modern knowledge, in fact, this was well established to be its biggest downfall in its early conception back in the early 1900s. Taking advantage of this vantage situation, yeast can fill the empty space, multiplying until they become a collective force that further exacerbates the dysbiosis[52].

Overconsumption of alcoholic beverages: Excessive consumption of alcohol is known to kill a multitude of useful bacteria in the digestive tract as well as overloading the liver. Alcohol is a yeast by-product, which can assist in the fuelling of fungal growth. It is possible for Candida to create alcohol as a by-product on consumption of sugar. In fact, individuals with Candida overgrowth have higher blood alcohol levels and can literally become drunk eating an excessive amount of sugar. It is also possible for someone to experience 'hangover' symptoms, potentially explaining issues with concentration, nausea and increased headaches.

Hormonal Imbalances: It is well known that women are more susceptible to Candida then men, this is believed to be caused by hormonal imbalances. During periods of hormonal change such as; menopause, the consumption of birth control pills or pregnancy, it is easier for the intestinal biome to be disrupted allowing the ever advantageous Candida to take control and boost growth.

Bowel problems: Conditions such as constipation, diarrhea, parasites, worms, IBS, leaky guy, heartburn, gas and bloating may trigger a Candida Overgrowth. Not only are these signs of a yeast infection, these can also help cause the problem. Almost like the "which came first, the chicken or the egg" dilemma. Anything that causes dysbiosis in the gut flora may also cause Candida overgrowth.

Others: A variety of other 'causes' that have been claimed. In fact, the list is almost inexhaustible. However, there is little scientific proof to back up these claims so take them with a grain of salt. Some examples are:

- Increased stress
- Oral contraceptives
- Environmental moulds or chemicals
- Toxic metals and food Chemicals

THE NO-NONSENSE GUIDE TO DIGESTIVE DISEASES

- Immune deficiency

The first step in self-diagnosis is matching the cause of the condition with current and previous actions. The next but equally important step is matching the symptoms currently experienced to confirmed Candida overgrowth symptoms.

HEALTHFUL PUBLICATIONS

The Symptoms Associated With Candida Overgrowth

Candida Overgrowth is a rare medical condition as its symptoms are not limited to the gut alone. As Candida can penetrate into the bloodstream, symptoms can spread throughout the body. This medical condition is often jointly presented with other associated medical conditions that are more defined in their manifestation.

Although the following list of symptoms isn't extensive, there are a few recurring symptoms shown in individuals with Candida Overgrowth.

Food Intolerance

Candida overgrowth is also a major cause of food allergies. Candida can exacerbate the intestines causing Leaky Gut Syndrome (or Intestinal Permeability). Leaky Gut Syndrome is a weakening and inflamed intestinal wall. This topic is explained thoroughly in the next

THE NO-NONSENSE GUIDE TO DIGESTIVE DISEASES

chapter. There are several factors that are responsible for this disorder. During Candida overgrowth, the yeast cells attach themselves to the intestinal walls of the digestive tract. This slowly weakens the lining of the intestines allowing Candida to penetrate the membrane and move into the bloodstream. The subsequent entry of food particles and Candida cells into the blood stream triggers a strong immune response, which will eventually lead to the inflammation of the intestinal wall.

The purpose of the immune system is to react and destroy any foreign body that enters the human bloodstream. During this process, the body's immune system produces antibodies that recognize these foreign bodies and trigger a secondary immune response. This hypersensitivity of the immune system is the origin of food allergies. The allergic responses are capable of mounting intense pressure on the adrenal glands as well as the body's immune system. Unfortunately, the adrenal glands and body's immune system are responsible for fighting off Candida. This means that Leaky Gut Syndrome can distract the immune system and adrenal glands, allowing a further rise in Candida Overgrowth. In order to avoid this, it is imperative that Leaky Gut Syndrome is controlled.

Digestion

The consumption of foods may cause the following digestive problems, it's important to make the distinction between if these problems are being caused by food in general or by specific foods. If the latter, it is wise to remove these problematic foods as further irritation to the stomach can exacerbate the problem.

- Chronic diarrhea, constipation or IBS
- Abdominal bloating, gas or distention
- Indigestion, cramps, gripping or discomfort

Overall Wellbeing

Patients with Autoimmune diseases like Multiple Sclerosis, Hashimoto's thyroiditis, Ulcerative colitis, Rheumatoid arthritis, Psoriasis and Lupus are at higher risk of obtaining an overgrowth. The leaking of particles into the bloodstream mean that these invasions can be fought by white blood cells at various locations of the body. This can cause a variety of

THE NO-NONSENSE GUIDE TO DIGESTIVE DISEASES

problems in specific or large areas depending on the intensity of the problem.

- Impaired immunity or frequent infections
- Chronic fatigue
- Fungal infections that can appear on the nails, skin or genitals
- Skin infections like eczema, hives, psoriasis or rashes
- Itchy ears

Mental effects

The loss of key nutrients may starve the brain of essential aid, allowing the onset of various conditions.

- Headaches or migraines
- Inability to concentrate and memory loss
- Irritability
- Depression, apathy, mood swings and irritability
- Strong cravings for sugar and refined carbohydrates

The symptom listed here are a broad set of conditions that have been attributed to this syndrome. As the field evolves and scientific research lends more evidence to it,

HEALTHFUL PUBLICATIONS

the symptoms associated with this condition will become more defined.

THE NO-NONSENSE GUIDE TO
DIGESTIVE DISEASES

Diagnosing Candida Overgrowth

Candida is extremely controversial. Many medical professionals fail to identity it as an independent illness, as a result, many patients have been unable to get relevant medical attention. The whole situation is further compounded by the fact that most of the symptoms associated with Candida Overgrowth can also be linked to several other illnesses.

1) Home-based test for Candida Overgrowth

Even though an increasing number of doctors claim to diagnose Candidiasis, coming across a doctor that is able to identify and treat this illness is exceptionally rare. Fortunately, there are a range of simple tests that prove to be moderately reliable at diagnosing Candidiasis at home.

Spittle Test: The spittle test is very simple. First thing in the morning, before brushing your teeth, you are required to fill a glass with bottled water and spit some saliva directly into it. After 20 minutes, come back and check the glass of water. Candida Overgrowth can be confirmed by the occurrence of any of the following:

- The presence of cloudy saliva at the bottom of the glass
- The suspension of opaque specks of saliva in the water
- Strings coming down through the water from the saliva resting at the top

This test isn't entirely reliable. Its main function is to determine the thickness of mucus. Unfortunately, there are many other factors that can boost the thickness of mucus; many of which are not related to Candida. People with allergies to dairy products or are dehydrated show a higher concentration of mucus. Therefore it's recommended to drink plenty of water the previous day, so as not to be dehydrated first thing in the morning.

2) Laboratory Tests

Even though diagnosis is difficult, there are reliable medical tests readily available. These tests vary in effectiveness.

THE NO-NONSENSE GUIDE TO DIGESTIVE DISEASES

Blood test: This is used to analyse the levels of IgG, IgA, and IgM (Candida anti-bodies) in the blood stream. The levels of these antibodies are typically proportionate to Candida overgrowth. In other words, high levels of these antibodies indicate an overgrowth of Candida. This test is the most reliable out of the three.

Urine Organix Dysbiosis Test: This test is specifically used to analyse the level of D-Arabinitol in the body. D-Arabinitol is one of the main waste products of Candida. High levels of D-Arabinitol in the body indicate the presence of Candida in the upper gut or small intestines. Also, the Urine Organix Dysbiosis Test can detect tartaric acid, which is another waste product of Candida yeast overgrowth. An elevated level of these waste products indicates an overgrowth of Candida. However, Urine Organix Dysbiosis Test is not as accurate as a blood test.

Stool testing: Stool testing is specifically used to determine which bacterial organism is flourishing in the digestive tract. One advantage of this test is that it can be used to determine specific species that exist in the digestive tract.

HEALTHFUL PUBLICATIONS

Note that there are two types of testing; a comprehensive and standard stool test. Unfortunately, stool testing can only be used to analyse the levels of yeast, pathogenic and friendly bacteria, it is not able to effectively analyse levels of Candida. Therefore, this test is the least reliable out of the three.

THE NO-NONSENSE GUIDE TO DIGESTIVE DISEASES

Your Treatment Plan

The process of eradicating Candida overgrowth is a long and perilous journey that requires a dedicated lifestyle change. This change will make you a healthier person, it'll even help to reduce weight. Simply put, three things need to happen. Firstly, Candida's main food supply needs to be replaced with foods that are antifungal in nature and attack Candida. Secondly, the specific form of Candidiasis needs to be treated if applicable. Finally we can aid the healing process with natural remedies. The restoration of friendly bacteria helps to keep future Candida growth rate in check, while the healing of the digestive tract helps to prevent Candida from gaining entry into the bloodstream.

Strict Diet Control – Cutting off Candida's food supply

This is by far the most important step; if you are only going to take one action, make sure it's this. The downside of a Candida diet is that it is extremely limiting, the upside is that this diet is in fact extremely healthy, not only curing Candida but granting a variety of other health benefits associated with it.

As previously mentioned, Candida feeds on carbohydrates and sugars. Therefore these need to be removed in practically all forms. This means eliminating:

- Sugary foods (honey, chocolate, syrup, artificial sweeteners etc.)
- Sugary fruits (fresh, dried or canned fruit. Fruit juice is extremely high in sugars)
- Alcohol (all forms as it is high in sugar and it temporarily weakens the immune system)
- High carb/starchy foods (wheat, rye, oats, barley, rice, potatoes, carrots, sweet potatoes, yams, parsnips, peas, beets and beans)
- Dairy products (milk, cream, cheese, whey products, etc. as these contain lactose; a natural sugar)
- Condiments (mayonnaise, ketchup, relish etc. as these all contain hidden sugars)

Some foods are known to suppress the immune system and others are loaded with additives that harm digestion. Eliminate these foods to fully support health regeneration:

THE NO-NONSENSE GUIDE TO DIGESTIVE DISEASES

• Pork and processed meats (pork is more harmful to a weakened digestive system than other meats while processed meats are packed with extra sugars and additives)
• High mould-content foods (nuts and mushrooms etc.)
• Fish (all fish are high in toxins and heavy metals. Wild salmon and sardines have lower levels of toxins so these are fine in moderation)
• Caffeine (coffee, tea, green tea, soda and energy drinks as these weaken the immune system by impairing adrenals)
• Yeast packed foods (vinegar, these foods cause further inflammation. Why add more yeast when trying to fight an intrusive yeast problem?)

Generally, it takes between three and six months to bring Candida growth back under control. However, a faster result can be obtained by supplementing the process with daily intake of anti-fungal medications like, Diflucan and Nyastatin. Be warmed though, doctors only prescribe fungal medications in extreme circumstances because of the damaging side effects that include; rashes, inflammation and allergic reactions. Alternatively, you can use a natural supplement called caprylic acid. Caprylic Acid is obtained from coconut oil and acts by "poking holes" in the yeast cell wall. The holes will eventually lead to the death of the yeast. Unlike some natural supplements, caprylic Acid doesn't kill good bacteria.

Substituting Candida Enhancing Foods for Candida Fighting Foods

There are some special foods that are particularly helpful in preventing Candida. The list is actually inexhaustible. Below are 10 helpful foods that help fight back against Candida.

Cayenne Pepper: Cayenne pepper supports the digestion process of the body. It also cleans up the bowel, thereby reducing constipation and body toxins. This helps to boost the body's immune system. Cayenne also facilitates the body metabolism and blood circulation, thereby eradicating fatigue, which is a main symptom of Candida.

Coconut Oil: This has antifungal properties. Coconut Oil is also capable of strengthening the immune system.

THE NO-NONSENSE GUIDE TO DIGESTIVE DISEASES

Garlic: Garlic is another wonderful substance that has strong antifungal properties. Thus, it's able to attack Candida.

Ginger: This is food substance is very effective in detoxifying the human internal system. In addition to this, ginger can also increase blood circulation.

Lemon and lime Juice: Juices obtained from lemon and limes have been found to stimulate the peristaltic action of the colon. Peristaltic action is solely responsible for getting things moving inside the digestive tract, cleansing along the way.

Olive Oil: Olive oil is another great anti-fungal substance. Its anti-fungal activities can be attributed to one of its constituent generally known as Oleuropein. In addition to this function, olive oil also has the capacity to balance blood sugar.

Onions: These exhibit strong anti-fungal, anti-parasitic and anti-bacterial activities. Therefore, they are very helpful in curtailing Candida Overgrowth.

Pumpkin Seeds: Pumpkin seeds are very rich in Omega-3 fatty acids. These unique acids also exhibit strong anti-fungal, anti-parasitic and anti-bacterial activities.

Raw Apple Cider Vinegar: This contains natural enzymes that encourage the growth of healthy bacteria, and maintain the pH level of the body. It is the only form of vinegar allowed.

Rutabaga: Despite its apparent starchy nature, this substance has very strong antifungal properties. Thus, it's recommended for anybody that hopes to check Candida overgrowth.

Specific Treatment

Before commencing treatment it is important that the type of Candidiasis has been properly diagnosed. If the Candida problem isn't severe enough to cause Candidiasis then this part can be skipped. Each type of Candidiasis has a specific treatment.

Treatment for Thrush and Invasive Candidiasis: Thrush has the potential to infect the bloodstream. It's a very serious illness and must be reported to the doctor immediately if it's been identified at home. The treatment method varies depending on three factors; overall health, age and severity of the infection. Thrush

THE NO-NONSENSE GUIDE TO DIGESTIVE DISEASES

and Invasive Candidiasis are treated with antifungal medicine which can be in mouthwash or pill forms. However, if the infection resists this treatment and subsequently become life threatening, it can then be treated with a powerful antifungal drug, administered through a vein (IV).

Treatment for Urino-genital Yeast Infection: This type of infection should be treated urgently to avoid passing it to a sexual partner. Currently, there are numerous over-the-counter drugs for treating yeast infections. They come in several forms; such as creams or suppositories that can be place inside the vagina or rubbed onto the penis. Most doctors recommend a single 150-milligram dose
of Diflucan (fluconazole) for patients that have never had vaginal yeast infection or are first time suffers of the disease. A reoccurring yeast infection can be treated with anti-fungal medicine. This medicine should first be administered every 10 to 14 days, and then once a week for six months. Boric acid capsules may also be recommended for up to two weeks.

Treatment for Leaky Gut Syndrome: This defect

is primarily controlled by a strict diet. In addition to reducing the population of Candida in the digestive tract, the Candida diet can also be used to restore the integrity of the intestinal walls. People that are having Candida-related food allergies should endeavour to avoid substances that are likely to increase the stress on their intestinal wall. Some examples of these include; laxatives, caffeine, spices etc. The intake of soluble fibre should also be encouraged. Generally, soluble fibres help to speed up the movement of waste through the intestine. This minimizes its chance of leaking into the bloodstream. Some good examples of fibre-rich meals include; oat bran, psyllium husks, dried beans and peas, raw vegetables etc. However it is important to tackle this stage after you have beaten Candida as a lot of foods beneficial to the gut are prohibited on a Candida diet. Leaky Gut Syndrome can also be controlled through rotation of food. This involves leaving a gap of a few days between a particular meal. This strategy helps to give to give the immune system a break and reduces the chance of building up extra intolerances.

Regenerating the Gut with Natural Remedies

THE NO-NONSENSE GUIDE TO DIGESTIVE DISEASES

There are natural remedies that can be used to treat Candida Overgrowth. These remedies come in a wide variety of forms which consists mainly of herbs and supplements.

Acidophilus: Acidophilus is a bacterium that is specifically helpful in removing Candida from the digestive tract. It executes this function by increasing the PH level of the intestinal tract, thereby making it too acidic for Candida growth. The effectiveness of this useful organism can be greatly facilitated by supplementing with a hydrogen peroxide-producing strain of the organism popularly known as DSS-1. DSS-1 is also helpful in reducing the incidence of antibiotic-induced yeast infections. Acidophilus helps to maintain the microbial balance that exists within the digestive tract.

Fibber: Good sources of soluble fibre can be found in flaxseed, psyllium husks, guar gum and pectin. Taking about one teaspoon to one tablespoon of soluble fibre from the above on an empty stomach is a very effective way of getting rid of Candida Overgrowth. The specified quantity of soluble fibre should be mixed in an 8 oz. glass of water and taken 2 times per day.

Enteric-coated essential oils: Taking enteric-coated capsules that consist of peppermint oil, oregano oil and other volatile oils can also restrict Candida Overgrowth. The intake of these highly effective oils should last for several months. A typical dosage is two capsules two times a day with water, make sure to take them in between meals. The liquid form of these oils should never be ingested as these volatile oils are highly toxic in nature. Therefore, it's not advisable to break the capsule before ingestion.

Enteric-coated garlic: Candia Overgrowth can also be prevented or even treated with enteric-coated garlic. Enteric-coated garlic is specially designed to open upon once it's reached the intestines. They can also be used simultaneously with volatile oils. A typical dose is one capsule two times per day.

THE NO-NONSENSE GUIDE TO DIGESTIVE DISEASES

Recent Advancements in Science

Science progresses on a daily basis, so much so that it is hard for general practitioners to keep up-to-date. It's important to note that this does not always mean new information is superior. In fact, studies that have plenty of counter-arguments or are used as a basis for further investigation are the most reliable. Although, it never hurts to stay one step ahead. This section summarises interesting advancements that have occurred in the last few years.

Redefining the threat of Candida

As we are already aware, there is very little research and recognition of Candida and how it impacts those that suffer from it. In fact, the severity of a Candida infection is a relatively new concept. This is evident in a 2014 research article by the Pravara Institute of Medical Sciences in India[53]. This article hopes to redefine the general association of Candida. It states and clearly defines that Candida can cause disabling and lethal infections.

Causation

The previous article calls candidiasis the "disease of the diseased"[53]. Further confirmation comes from a 2014 journal, stating something already covered, consuming antibiotics contributes to the overgrowth of Candida[54]. Not only this but a patient's own microbiota can influence and even cause Candida overgrowth.

Treatment

A journal published in 2016 focusing on how to advance the diagnosis and therapy of Candida contributes to the already mentioned scarce understanding[55]. It suggests areas that should be further explored, however, one interesting point is that dietary fermentable fibre (such as found in onion, leeks and garlic) increases the production of dendritic cells which support the immune system by capturing antigens and activating the immune response.

Natural fungicides such as SCFAs to combat skin based candida

THE NO-NONSENSE GUIDE TO DIGESTIVE DISEASES

The final article being investigated from the Journal of Microbial & Biochemical Technology links SCFAs or short chain fatty-acids as a new set of tools being used in medicines fighting fungal and bacterial based activity on the skin[56]. This is done by promoting probiotic activities of the skin that outcompete pathogens. Hopefully SCFAs will be used in more promising medicine in the future.

HEALTHFUL PUBLICATIONS

Conclusion

Candida is a family of fungal organisms that are naturally found within the human digestive tract. They exist in very small quantities and play very significant roles in digestion and subsequent absorption of nutrients from the digestive tract.

Although extremely beneficial, the overproduction of this fungal organism increases its ability to break down the wall of the intestine and allows it to penetrate the bloodstream. Once this occurs, the fungus is able to release toxic by-products into the internal system of the body, thereby giving rise to a disease condition generally known as Candidiasis. This disease is capable of affecting the skin, genitals, throat, mouth and even blood.

Although a variety of medicinal interventions can be taken that fights funguses, the most effective step in combatting this disorder is to amend diet and lifestyle. Therefore, if you are experiencing any

THE NO-NONSENSE GUIDE TO DIGESTIVE DISEASES

symptoms of Candida it's imperative to make healthy lifestyle changes to keep it in check and ultimately restore balance.

HEALTHFUL PUBLICATIONS

Leaky Gut Syndrome

"The digestive canal represents a tube passing through the entire organism and communicating with the external world, i.e. as it were the external surface of the body, but turned inwards and thus hidden" ~ Ivan Pavlov

What is Leaky Gut Syndrome?

The Gastrointestinal Tract (GIT) is a water-tight system compartmentalised within the core of the body. This system interacts with other bodily systems in a very controlled and precise manner. A healthy bowel (combination of small and large intestines) exchanges nutrients with the rest of the body, transferring them from within the cells lining the wall of the bowel into the blood stream and ultimately to the rest of the body. These cells, known as epithelial cells, are held together by tightly compacted proteins called desmosomes.

However, this water-tight system can malfunction, leading to a leakage of contents from within. It is theorised that individuals affected with Leaky Gut Syndrome (or Leaky Bowel Syndrome) inhibit loosely packed desmosomes which cause the lining of the bowel to become permeable[57]. This allows food particles to pass through the gap between these cells in an uncontrolled and dangerous manner.

The process of breaking down food throughout the GIT is precise, allowing only smaller nutrients (such as peptides/amino acids, sugars and lipids) to pass through into the blood stream. If the permeability of the gut is breached then macro nutrients that haven't been properly digested, waste that would otherwise be excreted and gut microflora will seep into the bloodstream[58]. Not only does this mean beneficial nutrients are not properly absorbed into the body, harmful substances are passed into circulation.

The human immune system constantly monitors activities that take place in the body. A unique, but vital feature of the immune system is its ability to distinguish between natural occurring processes and foreign activities. Since the intestines are an enclosed unit its contents are not exposed to the immune system. If the permeability of the intestines increases and particles pass through, the immune system identifies these particles as foreign and launches an immune response against them[59]. This interplay between the intestine and the immune system may explain why people with Leaky Gut Syndrome complain about additional food sensitivities[60]. As contents from the gut are leaked into the blood stream the immune system reacts by creating anti-bodies developed to combat these 'foreign' particles, meaning, next time that food is eaten, these anti-bodies will react against them. These food sensitivities can present themselves in the form of hives, eczema and other irritating symptoms[61].

HEALTHFUL PUBLICATIONS

What Causes Leaky Gut Syndrome?

The medical community have not been able to reach a consensus on the underlying causes of this disorder. However, more and more scientific evidence is showing that factors such as diet[62], chronic stress[63], certain medications[64] and bacterial imbalance are the key contributing factors that lead to the development of Leaky Gut Syndrome.

The interplay between other digestive diseases and Leak Gut Syndrome aren't entirely understood. There is often debate whether something causes intestinal permeability or if intestinal permeability is the cause[60]. This cause-or-effect list includes food allergies, inflammatory bowel disease, celiac disease and even type 1 diabetes[60].

An excessive intake of alcohol is also considered one of the most common causes of Leaky Gut Syndrome[65]. This is a simplification but the message is the same, it's important to keep alcohol consumption levels under control

THE NO-NONSENSE GUIDE TO DIGESTIVE DISEASES

if intestinal permeability is being monitored. Alcohol promotes the growth of Gram negative bacteria (a specific group of bacteria which includes E. coli & chlamydia etc.), which creates an accumulation of endotoxins (toxins within bacteria). Alcohol metabolism by Gram negative bacteria and intestinal epithelial cells (cells lining the oesophagus) promotes the accumulated growth of acetaldehyde (group 1 carcinogenic), which increases intestinal permeability to these endotoxins.

Most of today's research points to the influence of a class of medicines called non-steroidal anti-inflammatory drugs (NSAIDs) in the creation of a leaky gut[66]. Common examples of this class of drug include pain killers such as aspirin and ibuprofen that are easily available over-the-counter in pharmacies. Research shows that NSAIDs damage the proteins that hold cells together in the intestine. This results in increased permeability of the gut wall.

As well as NSAIDs, there is growing evidence that certain antibiotic strains contribute to this condition[67]. The gut microflora contains billions of thriving micro-organisms, most of them being beneficial to us. However, there are certain species of organisms that, though beneficial, need to be kept in-check by other organisms. There is a constant competition between these good and bad organisms inside the gut, luckily our system favours the good microbes. When we ingest antibiotics, they kill gut micro-organisms in a non-selective manner which often leads to an imbalance between good and bad microbes, a phenomenon called dysbiosis. Taking advantage of this vantage situation bad microbes can multiply, causing the immune system to react. A stimulated immune system can lead to inflammation, damaging the integrity of the intestinal wall and acting as a contributing factor to Leaky Gut Syndrome[68]. It's possible for antibiotics taken early in childhood to have negative repercussions within our gut later in life[69].

Leaky Gut Syndrome can contribute to the development of other medical conditions such as Crohn's disease – a chronic intestinal disorder that affects millions globally[70]. The following conditions are also thought to be triggered by Intestinal permeability (Leaky Gut)

THE NO-NONSENSE GUIDE TO DIGESTIVE DISEASES

or the cause of it:

- Coeliac Disease[71]
- Irritable Bowel Disease[72]
- Infections of the intestines – such as the norovirus and giardiasis[73]
- Chronic Kidney Disease[74]
- HIV/AIDS[73]
- Cystic Fibrosis[75]
- Type 1 Diabetes[76]

Coeliac disease is of special importance; a condition characterised by hyper-sensitivity to wheat, barley and rye protein gluten[77]. Physicians often check for coeliac disease in individuals that exhibit similar symptoms as Leaky Gut Syndrome and luckily, coeliac disease is easier to identify. Patients with Coeliac disease create antibodies that seek to destroy a substance in gluten called gliadin. The antibodies then cause the lining of the gut to become inflamed, further increasing chances of leaky gut syndrome[71]. Patients that suffer both conditions will not fully recover by removing gluten alone, they will also have to treat their harder to diagnose Leaky Gut.

Leaky Gut Syndrome can be caused by a

variety of other conditions, worsening over time until these triggers are dealt with. This can create a circular effect. For example, individuals affected with conditions such as eczema, asthma or urticarial exhibit a higher level of intestinal permeability[78]. When these individuals are exposed to foods that they are sensitive to, inflammation occurs, which aggravates the existing eczema or urticarial as well as further increasing intestinal permeability, making all conditions worse.

THE NO-NONSENSE GUIDE TO
DIGESTIVE DISEASES

The Symptoms Associated with Leaky Gut Syndrome

Leaky Gut is a complicated medical condition as its symptoms are not limited to the gut alone. Particles ingested, as well as ordinary bacterial inhabitants of the gut can penetrate into the bloodstream causing symptoms to spread throughout the body[58]. This medical condition is often jointly presented with other associated medical conditions that are more defined in their manifestation.

Although the list of following symptoms isn't extensive, there are a few recurring symptoms shown in individuals with leaky gut.

Digestion

The consumption of food may cause the following digestive problems, however, it is important to identify whether these problems are being caused by food in general or by particular food or food groups. If the latter is the case, it is wise to remove these problematic foods as further irritation to the stomach can exacerbate the problem.

- Food sensitivities or Allergies[61]
- Chronic diarrhoea, constipation or IBS[72]
- Abdominal bloating, gas or distention[72]
- Indigestion, cramps, gripping or discomfort[72]

Overall Wellbeing

When particles leak into the bloodstream, white blood cells can fight these invasions at various locations within the body. This can cause a variety of problems in small or large areas depending on the concentration of particles leaked.

- Impaired immunity or frequent infections[73]
- Joint pain, muscle weakness or exercise intolerance[79]
- Skin rashes, irritation or eruptions (acne or boils)[61]

Mental effects

The loss of key nutrients may limit the brain of essential aid allowing various conditions to manifest.

THE NO-NONSENSE GUIDE TO DIGESTIVE DISEASES

The Symptoms Associated with Leaky Gut Syndrome

Leaky Gut is a complicated medical condition as its symptoms are not limited to the gut alone. Particles ingested, as well as ordinary bacterial inhabitants of the gut can penetrate into the bloodstream causing symptoms to spread throughout the body[58]. This medical condition is often jointly presented with other associated medical conditions that are more defined in their manifestation.

Although the list of following symptoms isn't extensive, there are a few recurring symptoms shown in individuals with leaky gut.

Digestion

The consumption of food may cause the following digestive problems, however, it is important to identify whether these problems are being caused by food in general or by particular food or food groups. If the latter is the case, it is wise to remove these problematic foods as further irritation to the stomach can exacerbate the problem.

- Food sensitivities or Allergies[61]
- Chronic diarrhoea, constipation or IBS[72]
- Abdominal bloating, gas or distention[72]
- Indigestion, cramps, gripping or discomfort[72]

Overall Wellbeing

When particles leak into the bloodstream, white blood cells can fight these invasions at various locations within the body. This can cause a variety of problems in small or large areas depending on the concentration of particles leaked.

- Impaired immunity or frequent infections[73]
- Joint pain, muscle weakness or exercise intolerance[79]
- Skin rashes, irritation or eruptions (acne or boils)[61]

Mental effects

The loss of key nutrients may limit the brain of essential aid allowing various conditions to manifest.

THE NO-NONSENSE GUIDE TO DIGESTIVE DISEASES

for mannitol is about 14% while less than 1% of lactulose is usually absorbed. All of the mannitol and lactulose absorbed is excreted.

The patient is given this solution and urine samples are then analysed after 6 hours to check for the content of mannitol and lactulose. Possible diagnoses made on the results are as follows:

a) Low levels of both Mannitol and lactulose: Such a situation would indicate malabsorption as mannitol is a small molecule and is easily absorbed through the intestinal lining into the blood stream. A low level of mannitol in the urine would indicate that there is malabsorption.

b) Elevated levels of both Mannitol and Lactulose: Such a result would point towards increased intestinal permeability and a high possibility of a leaky gut.

Stool Sample Analysis

Another test that assesses the permeability of the gut is a stool sample analysis[81]. Stool sample analysis shows how well macronutrients are absorbed into the body by analysing the macronutrient contents of stool. Leaky gut syndrome also alters the composition of gut microflora in the stool sample. Hence, it is important for this parameter to be checked.

Testing for Food Sensitivities and Allergies

One of the most common symptoms that patients with leaky gut syndrome exhibit is increased sensitivity to foods that they were once fine with consuming. In order to confirm these sensitivities doctors usually suggest allergy testing. There are a few ways to test for food sensitivities:

a) **Skin Prick Test**: The skin prick test is one of the most common ways of identifying sensitivities to substances[82]. The test is usually performed on the back or the forearm and takes about 20-30 minutes, it also allows the patient to discuss results almost immediately with the doctor. In this test, the doctor places a drop of fluid containing the allergen on the surface of the skin. When being checked for food allergies, food components such as lactose are used. After placing the drop of allergen on the skin, the area is pricked with a sterile lancet

THE NO-NONSENSE GUIDE TO DIGESTIVE DISEASES

or scratched so as to push the allergen inside the body. When this happens, and if the person is indeed allergic to that food substance, the immune system reacts causing inflammation, redness and making it sore.

Skin prick tests may be slightly uncomfortable but are usually well-tolerated. The local itch and swelling is reversible and the itching subsides in a couple of hours. In case the swelling persists, there are treatments available which allow the site to be easily treated.

b) **Patch Test**: A patch test is also frequently used by doctors to assess sensitivities to food[83]. Such a test is specifically recommended to individuals that are suspected of having allergic contact dermatitis and/or atopic dermatitis, a condition that makes the patient react to metals or cosmetic preservatives. In this test, multiple allergens can be treated at one time. This patch is pressed onto the individual's back and the reaction is monitored for about 48 hours.

c) **Radioallergosorbent Test (RAST):** The RAST is a blood test that measures immune hypersensitivities[84]. While skin tests are usually used, RAST and other blood based allergic tests are used when individuals are suffering from skin conditions such as severe eczema or if an individual is taking medications (such as antihistamines) that can interfere with accurate skin prick testing.

Amino Acid Analysis

Amino acids are the building blocks of proteins, which are one of the most important macromolecules in the body[85]. Amino acids and proteins are required to carry out tissue maintenance activities, producing enzymes, antibodies and many other biological functions. However, there are about 8 different amino acids that the body cannot make on its own and is dependent on dietary sources. These amino acids are essential and play a key role in maintaining the integrity of the immune system.

Healthcare practitioners may suggest amino acid analysis for patients with suspected leaky gut syndrome. This analysis allows a physician to assess the overall physical well-being of the individual and allows insight into possible symptoms of chronic fatigue associated with Leaky Gut Syndrome.

HEALTHFUL PUBLICATIONS

Your 4 Step Treatment Plan

As Leaky Gut Syndrome is still yet to gain a high level of interest by the medical community its treatment options are limited. However, the condition is indeed treatable, so long as the individual follows a strict procedure and puts their full attention into curing Leaky Gut Syndrome. As with most diseases affecting the gut, treatment methodologies are largely centred on strict dieting with support from medicines and supplements. Individuals diagnosed with Leaky Gut should adhere to the following dos and do not's when it comes to diet:

Do's

1) Eat fruits and vegetables grown organically that help fight inflammation. Tomatoes, strawberries, blueberries, cherries, oranges and green leafy vegetables such as spinach, kale or collards are naturally anti-inflammatory[86].

2) Make sure to get plenty of Essential Fatty

THE NO-NONSENSE GUIDE TO DIGESTIVE DISEASES

Acids. The human body cannot create these types of fatty acids. These are normally obtained from foods such as Sunflower, safflower, wheat germ, sesame etc. Essential fatty acids have anti-oxidant properties and help to improve immune function of the body as well as countering inflammation[87].

3) Consume garlic & turmeric for their anti-oxidant and immune boosting properties[86].

Do not's

1) Check the ingredients list on food packaging to avoid ingredients that you are sensitive to[61].

2) Keep an eye on your digestion after consuming the 8 most common food allergens, which are required to be defined by law in some countries (such as the US) on the packaging of foods. These are; milk, eggs, peanuts, tree nuts (almonds, cashews etc.), fish, shellfish, soy and wheat.

3) In 2008 alcohol was scientifically proven to increase intestinal permeability[65]. Reduce intake as much as possible.

4) Fizzy drink consumption should be monitored as they contain a high amount of fructose which can increase permeability[88].

5) Monitor external stimuli, such as cosmetic and personal care products. Under a physiological state such as leaky gut, the immune system is hypersensitive, exposure to such synthetic chemicals have a higher chance of causing an allergic reaction such as rashes[89].

The following 4 step action plan is a commonly used tool physicians advise when an individual presents himself themselves with Leaky Gut Syndrome. This treatment flow is called the "Four R Program" based on its steps; Remove, Repair, Replace and Re-inoculate:

1) Remove

When a patient first presents his or her self to a doctor, it is common for the individual to succumb to increased stress due to this medical condition. Hence, the first step towards effective management of this condition to stabilise the patient and ease the distress. Such individuals are advised detox programs wherein potential allergens such as gluten, alcohol, caffeine and dairy products are strictly prohibited. This detox program helps the patient to stabilise and allows an easier diagnosis of potential allergens that may be responsible for increased intestinal permeability[86,87].

2) Replace

After the individual has stabilised, it is important that alternative foods are identified that help the individual to meet daily nutritional requirement, whilst avoiding irritants that affect the gut lining. Foods such as digestive herbs, digestive enzymes and probiotics[90]. Such foods give the intestine time to heal. It is the physician's responsibility to help the patient chart out a diet plan that suits the individual's specific needs.

3) Re-inoculate

As noted earlier, bacterial imbalance or dysbiosis is considered to be one of the leading triggers that result in Leaky Gut Syndrome. Dysbiosis results when an intake of medicine, such as antibiotics, cause a non-specific killing of gut microbes. Taking advantage of this situation unfriendly microbes out-grow their friendly counterparts and cause inflammation. It is essential to re-balance this delicate system. While probiotics are commonly prescribed in such condition, fermented and easy to metabolise foods such as curd may also be prescribed by physicians on a case-to-case basis. Consuming foods with high-fibre content can also help to re-establish gut microflora[91].

4) Repair

There are therapeutic options available that can help to rebuild the intestinal lining. Some of these therapies are as follows:

a) Epidermal Growth Factor (EGF) – Is a protein which has been shown to prevent Giardia lamblia from causing abnormalities in the intestinal junctions[92].

b) Saccharomyces boulardii – *S.boulardii* is a friendly strain of yeast whose beneficial effects on the gut are well demonstrated. It is widely used in the treatment of diarrhoea and in prevention and treatment of *Clostridium difficile* infections[93].

c) Lactobacillus caseii – Like *S.boulardii*, *Lactobacillus caseii* is also proven to help in the prevention and treatment of *Clostridium difficile* infection. The effects of *L.caseii* in improving the guts hyper permeability are clinically proven[94].

d) Glutamine and Glutathione – Glutamine and its derivative amino acid Glutathione are the human body's key defence mechanism against oxidative stress caused by inflammation. These amino acids use their anti-oxidant properties and help curb oxygen free-radicals that are produced during the process of inflammation. Glutamine and glutathione have been observed to aid in the regeneration of intestinal gut lining in patients that report damage to the gut lining, specifically post-exposure to chemotherapy or radiation therapy[95].

Diet plays a central role in the treatment and management of individuals with Leaky Gut Syndrome. The existing treatment options are focussed on managing diet so as to regulate the content of key nutrients such as amino acids, essential fatty acids and other anti-oxidants in the body. It is essential that after

HEALTHFUL PUBLICATIONS

recovering, the individual must adhere to healthy food and life-style habits so as to avoid relapse. As more research is conducted in this field increasing amounts of therapeutic options will become available.

THE NO-NONSENSE GUIDE TO DIGESTIVE DISEASES

Recent Advancements in Science

Science progresses on a daily basis, so much so that it is hard for general practitioners to keep up-to-date. It's important to note that this does not always mean new information is superior. In fact, studies that have plenty of counter-arguments or are used as a basis for further investigation are the most reliable. Although, it never hurts to stay one step ahead. This section summarises interesting advancements that have occurred in the last few years.

The Conception of Leaky Gut Syndrome

The first study is a review of recent scientific articles and papers. This review aims at evaluating the current definition of the Leaky Gut concept and whether it's merely fiction[96]. The conclusion from this paper is to resist the urge of linking gastrointestinal disorders with intestinal barrier dysfunction as there haven't been enough experiments to provide consistent supporting data. This review references a paper stating a certain amount of intestinal permeability is insufficient to cause disease[97]. However, it does state that "permeability can predispose and contribute to pathogenesis and progression of colitis and suggest that the same may be true in human IBD". This direct quote seems to contradict the conclusion of this paper. Unfortunately this means a lot more time is required until 'Leaky Gut Syndrome' has been proved and widely accepted among the science community.

Cause - Microflora

More studies are backing the idea that the microbiota directly influences day-to-day function[98]. It cements the fact that a diverse microbiota supports general health and wellbeing, but also that the lack of diversity can be a key factor in the development of diseases. This review also suggests that the diagnosis of a patient's microbiota can result in the detection of gut-related diseases, far before conventional methods can.

Diagnosis

The current diagnosis of Leaky Gut is mentioned

in a prior chapter. This next published article aims at defining a uniform method of detection[99]. More and more microbial products are using bacterial DNA in blood to detect intestinal permeability. This is a positive outcome as an effective and uniform method should be adopted, however, this article hints strongly towards measuring plasma endotoxin levels as it is more simple, making it easier to adopt.

Gut & Brain Connection

Interestingly, this area has received the most attention, perhaps due to the worlds shifting focus towards mental health. We already know that intestinal permeability influences mental health in a variety of ways; ranging from headaches to even depression[59]. Emerging theories suggest that intestinal permeability can lead to much more severe disorders like Alzheimer's disease[100]. The most current hypothesis behind Alzheimer's is that neuroinflammation and neurodegeneration are the main triggers. This review article shows an unreliable correlation between gut bacteria dysbiosis and Alzheimer's. It also heavily insists that there are a multitude of other tests that need to take place before the results of this article are taken seriously.

There are further studies reiterating the gut-brain axis and its importance in day-to-day mental wellbeing[101]. This next study suggests probiotics and prebiotics has antidepressant properties and should be taken alongside therapeutic treatment.

Possible Treatments

As of today, there is no drug commonly used to reduce intestinal permeability[102]. A peer-reviewed research article investigates if Lubiprostone, a drug used to combat chronic constipation, can potentially make an impact. 28 men were lactose – mannitol tested, given lubiprostone for a month and tested again. The results showed roughly a 40% decrease in the lactulose-mannitol level. However, blood endotoxin levels showed no significant change. Lubiprostone has a variety of side effects including nausea, vomiting, abdominal pain and diarrhea. This study suggests an interesting hypothesis which requires in-depth testing, counter-testing and analysis.

THE NO-NONSENSE GUIDE TO DIGESTIVE DISEASES

Recoflavone, otherwise known as DA-6034 is a derivative of a flavonoid; a plant based chemical that contributes to the vivid colours of fruits and vegetables[103]. The original flavonoid in question is called Eupatilin which comes from a plant called Artemisia asiatica. This plant belongs to the same daisy specie as mugwort, sagebrush and wormwood. DA-6034 is known for its anti-inflammatory properties for those suffering with inflammatory bowel disease. This journal investigates if DA-6034 can directly reduce intestinal permeability. The results were interesting but limited, they show the potential for preventing further intestinal permeability caused by NSAIDS but not in the reduction in permeability itself.

HEALTHFUL PUBLICATIONS

Conclusion

Leaky Gut Syndrome is a chronic medical condition affecting the gut. As of today the medical community is divided in acknowledging its existence, diagnosis and treatment. Intestinal permeability on the other hand has been studied in relation to a variety of other health issues, providing much of the sources contained within this book.

It is hypothesised that Leaky Gut Syndrome is caused by continued damage to the intestinal lining. Factors such as alcohol, food that the patient is sensitive to and medications such as NSAIDs (aspirin, ibuprofen etc.) are considered to be key triggers in the onset of this condition. There is also strong evidence that antibiotics create increased intestinal permeability. Antibiotics are said to cause dysbiosis, creating an imbalance in the microbial flora in the gut leading to inflammation that compromises the compactness of the intestinal wall.

Certain diagnosis tests can help confirm

the presence and identify the severity of this disease. A frequently employed diagnostic tool is the lactulose- mannitol test that checks for the permeability of sugars by assessing their concentrations six-hours after consumption via urine sample. If the lactulose – mannitol ratio is higher than 0.03, this indicates high intestinal permeability.

The treatment of Leaky Gut Syndrome focuses largely around effective diet management. Individuals that have this condition should follow a strict diet plan that ensures gut inflammation is brought down and intestinal repair is aided. Individuals with Leaky Gut Syndrome should keep away from irritants such as alcohol, NSAID drugs and antibiotics. The treatment of leaky gut is tough but possible. Physicians play an important part in creating bespoke diet plans and aiding in long term health.

HEALTHFUL PUBLICATIONS

Sources

[1] Klarenbeek, Bastiaan R., Niels de Korte, Donald L. van der Peet, and Miguel A. Cuesta. "Review of current classifications for diverticular disease and a translation into clinical practice." *International journal of colorectal disease* 27, no. 2 (2012): 207-214.

[2] Parks, T. G. "Diet and diverticular disease." *Proceedings of the Royal Society of Medicine* 67, no. 10 (1974): 1037.

[3] Diverticular Disease and Diverticulitis. NHS, 11 May 2005. Web. 15 Oct. 2014. www.nhs.uk/conditions/Diverticular-disease-and-Diverticulitis/Pages/Introduction.aspx

[4] Logan, Barry K., and Alan Wayne Jones. "Endogenous ethanol 'auto-brewery syndrome' as a drunk-driving defence challenge." Medicine, Science and the Law 40.3 (2000): 206-215.

[5] Diverticulosis and Diverticulitis. Better Health Channel. 1 June 2012. Web. 15 Oct. 2014. www.betterhealth.vic.gov.au/bhcv2/bhcarticles.nsf/pages/Diverticulosis_and_Diverticulitis.

[6] National Digestive Diseases Information Clearinghouse (NDDIC). Diverticular Disease. National Digestive Diseases Information Clearinghouse, 1 Sept. 2013. Web. 15 Oct. 2014. http://digestive.niddk.nih.gov/ddiseases/pubs/Diverticulosis/index.aspx.

[7] De Punder, Karin, and Leo Pruimboom. "The dietary intake of wheat and other cereal grains and their

role in inflammation." *Nutrients* 5, no. 3 (2013): 771-787.

[8] Bjarnason I., Hayllar J., MacPherson A. J. and Russell A. S. Department of Clinical Biochemistry, King's College School of Medicine and Dentistry, London, England.
Gastroenterology 104(6):1832-1847 (1993).

[9] Collins S. M. American Journal of Physiology - Gastrointestinal and Liver Physiology. March 2001, 280 (3) G315-G318 (1993).

[10] Candela, M. et al. Interaction of probiotic Lactobacillus and Bifidobacterium strains with human intestinal epithelial cells: adhesion properties, competition against enteropathogens and modulation of IL-8 production. Int. J. Food Microbiol. 125, 286–292 (2008).

[11] Fukuda, S. et al. Bifidobacteria can protect from enteropathogenic infection through production of acetate. Nature 469, 543–547 (2011).

[12] Sonnenburg, J. L. et al. Glycan foraging in vivo by an intestine-adapted bacterial symbiont. Science 307, 1955–1959 (2005).

[13] Yatsunenko, T. et al. Human gut microbiome viewed across age and geography. Nature 486, 222–227 (2012).

[14] Olszak, T. et al. Microbial exposure during early life has persistent effects on natural killer T cell function. Science 336, 489–493 (2012).

[15] Cryan, J. F. et al. Mind-altering microorganisms: the impact of the gut microbiota on brain and behaviour. Nature Reviews Neuroscience 12, 701-

HEALTHFUL PUBLICATIONS

712 (2012).

[16] Soetan, Kehinde Olugboyega, and Charles Ojo Olaiya. "Summarizing Evidence Based Information on the Medical Importance of Dietary Fibre."*Annals of Food Science and Technology* 14, no. 2 (2013): 393-399.
[17] Aldoori, Walid H., Edward L. Giovannucci, Eric B. Rimm, Alvin L. Wing, Dimitrios V. Trichopoulos, and Walter C. Willett. "A prospective study of diet and the risk of symptomatic diverticular disease in men." *The American journal of clinical nutrition* 60, no. 5 (1994): 757-764.
[18] Aldoori, Walid, and Milly Ryan-Harshman. "Preventing diverticular disease. Review of recent evidence on high-fibre diets." *Canadian family physician* 48.10 (2002): 1632-1637.
[19] Floch, Martin H. "A hypothesis: is Diverticulitis a type of inflammatory bowel disease?." *Journal of clinical gastroenterology* 40 (2006): S121-S125.
[20] Martin, Sean T., and Luca Stocchi. "New and emerging treatments for the prevention of recurrent Diverticulitis." *Clinical and experimental gastroenterology*4 (2011): 203.
[21] Campbell, K., and R. J. C. Steele. "Non-steroidal anti-inflammatory drugs and complicated diverticular disease: A case—control study." *British journal of surgery* 78.2 (1991): 190-191.
[22] Kellow, J. E., et al. "Effects of acute psychologic stress on small-intestinal motility in health and the

THE NO-NONSENSE GUIDE TO DIGESTIVE DISEASES

irritable bowel syndrome." *Scandinavian journal of gastroenterology* 27.1 (1992): 53-58.

[23] Kvasnovsky, Charlotte Louise, and Savvas Papagrigoriadis. "Symptoms in patients with diverticular disease should not be labelled as IBS."*International journal of colorectal disease* 7, no. 30 (2015): 995-995.

[24] Jung, Sungmo, Hyuk Lee, Hyunsoo Chung, Jun Chul Park, Sung Kwan Shin, Sang Kil Lee, and Yong Chan Lee. "Incidence and predictive factors of irritable bowel syndrome after acute diverticulitis in Korea." *International journal of colorectal disease* 29, no. 11 (2014): 1369-1376.

[25] Tursi, Antonio, Walter Elisei, Marcello Picchio, Gian M. Giorgetti, and Giovanni Brandimarte. "Moderate to severe and prolonged left lower-abdominal pain is the best symptom characterizing symptomatic uncomplicated diverticular disease of the colon: a comparison with fecal calprotectin in clinical setting." *Journal of clinical gastroenterology* 49, no. 3 (2015): 218-221.

[26] Lahner, Edith, Cristina Bellisario, Cesare Hassan, Angelo Zullo, Gianluca Esposito, and Bruno Annibale. "Probiotics in the Treatment of Diverticular Disease. A Systematic." *J Gastrointestin Liver Dis* 25, no. 1 (2016): 79-86.

[27] McGuire HH, Jr, Haynes BW, Jr. Massive hemorrhage for diverticulosis of the colon: guidelines for therapy based on bleeding patterns

observed in fifty cases. Ann Surg. 1972;175:847–85.

[28] Nagata, Naoyoshi, Ryota Niikura, Takuro Shimbo, Naoki Ishizuka, Kazuyoshi Yamano, Kyoko Mizuguchi, Junichi Akiyama, Mikio Yanase, Masashi Mizokami, and Naomi Uemura. "High-dose barium impaction therapy for the recurrence of colonic diverticular bleeding: a randomized controlled trial." *Annals of surgery* 261, no. 2 (2015): 269-275.

[29] Fujihara, Shintaro, Hirohito Mori, Hideki Kobara, Noriko Nishiyama, Maki Ayaki, Toshiaki Nakatsu, and Tsutomu Masaki. "Use of an over-the-scope clip and a colonoscope for complete hemostasis of a duodenal diverticular bleed." *Endoscopy* 47, no. S 01 (2015): E236-E237.

[30] Lasser, Robert B., John H. Bond, and Michael D. Levitt. "The role of intestinal gas in functional abdominal pain." *New England Journal of Medicine* 293, no. 11 (1975): 524-526.

[31] NHS. Hypochondria. [ONLINE] Available at: http://www.nhs.uk/conditions/hypochondria/Pages/Introduction.aspx. [Last Accessed 23rd November 2014].

[32] Spiller, R. et al. Guidelines on the irritable bowel syndrome: mechanisms and practical management. *Gut*, *56*(12), 1770-1798 (2007).

[33] Yao, X. et al. Subtypes of irritable bowel syndrome on Rome III criteria: a multicenter study. *Journal of*

gastroenterology and hepatology, *27*(4), 760-765 (2012).

[34] NHS. *Irritable bowel syndrome (IBS) - Causes*. [ONLINE] Available at: http://www.nhs.uk/Conditions/Irritable-bowel-syndrome/Pages/Causes.aspx. [Last Accessed 28th November 2014] (2014).

[35] Konturek. S. J. et al. Brain-gut axis in pancreatic secretion and appetite control. J Physiol Pharmacol. 2003 Sep;54(3):293-317.

[36] Halpert, A., et al. What patients know about irritable bowel syndrome (IBS) and what they would like to know. National Survey on Patient Educational Needs in IBS and development and validation of the Patient Educational Needs Questionnaire (PEQ). *The American journal of gastroenterology*, *102*(9), 1972-1982 (2007).

[37] Hungin, A. P. S., et al. Irritable bowel syndrome in the United States: prevalence, symptom patterns and impact. *Alimentary pharmacology & therapeutics*, *21*(11), 1365-1375 (2005).

[38] Shepherd, S. J., et al. Dietary triggers of abdominal symptoms in patients with irritable bowel syndrome: randomized placebo-controlled evidence. *Clinical Gastroenterology and Hepatology*, *6*(7), 765-771 (2008).

[39] Friedrich, M., Grady, S. E., & Wall, G. C. (2010).

Effects of antidepressants in patients with irritable bowel syndrome and comorbid depression. *Clinical therapeutics*, *32*(7), 1221-1233.

[40] Lackner, J. M., Quigley, B. M., & Blanchard, E. B. (2004). Depression and abdominal pain in IBS patients: the mediating role of catastrophizing. *Psychosomatic medicine*, *66*(3), 435-441.

[41] Parlett, T. *Suitable products for the low FODMAP diet* [Brochure]. London, England: Department of Gastroenterology Department of Nutrition & Dietetics Guy's & St Thomas' NHS Foundation Trust London UK (2014).

[42] Rajilić-Stojanović, Mirjana, Daisy M. Jonkers, Anne Salonen, Kurt Hanevik, Jeroen Raes, Jonna Jalanka, Willem M. De Vos et al. "Intestinal Microbiota And Diet in IBS: Causes, Consequences, or Epiphenomena&quest." *The American journal of gastroenterology* 110, no. 2 (2015): 278-287.

[43] Jalanka, Jonna, Anne Salonen, Susana Fuentes, and Willem M. de Vos. "Microbial signatures in post-infectious irritable bowel syndrome–toward patient stratification for improved diagnostics and treatment." *Gut microbes* 6, no. 6 (2015): 364-369.

[44] Zhang, Yan, Lixiang Li, Chuanguo Guo, Dan Mu, Bingcheng Feng, Xiuli Zuo, and Yanqing Li. "Effects of probiotic type, dose and treatment duration on irritable bowel syndrome diagnosed by Rome III criteria: a meta-analysis."*BMC gastroenterology* 16, no. 1 (2016): 62.

[45] Nanayakkara, Wathsala S., Paula ML Skidmore, Leigh O'Brien, Tim J. Wilkinson, and Richard B.

THE NO-NONSENSE GUIDE TO DIGESTIVE DISEASES

Gearry. "Efficacy of the low FODMAP diet for treating irritable bowel syndrome: the evidence to date." *Clinical and Experimental Gastroenterology* 9 (2016): 131.
[46] Lozupone, C. A. et al. Diversity, stability and resilience of the human gut microbiota. Nature 489, 220-230 (2012).

[47] Mc Cullough, M. The Bottom Line on Soy and Breast Cancer Risk (2012).
http://www.cancer.org/cancer/news/expertvoices/post/2012/08/02/the-bottom-line-on-soy-and-breast-cancer-risk.aspx.
[48] Jackson, R. L., Greiwe, J. S. & Schwen, R. J. Emerging evidence of the health benefits of S-equol, an estrogen receptor beta agonist. Nutr. Rev. 69, 432–448 (2011).
[49] Biagi, E. et al. Through ageing, and beyond: gut microbiota and inflammatory status in seniors and centenarians. PLoS ONE 5, e10667 (2010).
[50] Manolakaki, D. et al. Candida infection and colonization among trauma patients. Virulence, 1(5), 367-375 (2010).
[51] Segal, E. Candida, still number one—what do we know and where are we going from
there? Mycoses, 48(s1), 3-11 (2005).
[52] Kennedy, M. J. et al. Mechanisms of association of Candida albicans with intestinal mucosa. Med Microbiol, 24, 333-341 (2005).
[53] Goyal, Rahul Kumar, Hiba Sami, Vashishth Mishra, Rajesh Bareja, and Rabindra Nath Behara. "Non-

HEALTHFUL PUBLICATIONS

Albicans Candiduria: An Emerging Threat." *Journal of Applied Pharmaceutical Science* 6, no. 3 (2016): 048-050.
[54] Guinea, J. "Global trends in the distribution of Candida species causing candidemia." *Clinical Microbiology and Infection* 20, no. s6 (2014): 5-10.

[55] Smeekens, S. P., F. L. van de Veerdonk, and M. G. Netea. "An Omics Perspective on Candida Infections: Toward Next-Generation Diagnosis and Therapy." *Frontiers in microbiology* 7 (2016).
[56] Kao, Ming-Shan, Yanhan Wang, Shinta Marito, Stephen Huang, Wan-Zhen Lin, Jon A. Gangoiti, Bruce A. Barshop et al. "The mPEG-PCL Copolymer for Selective Fermentation of Staphylococcus lugdunensis Against Candida parapsilosis in the Human Microbiome." *Journal of Microbial & Biochemical Technology* 8, no. 4 (2016): 259-265.
[57] Michielan, Andrea, and Renata D'Incà. "Intestinal permeability in inflammatory bowel disease: pathogenesis, clinical evaluation, and therapy of leaky gut." *Mediators of inflammation* 2015 (2015).
[58] Wyatt, Douglas A. "Leaky Gut Syndrome: A Modern Epidemic with an Ancient Solution?." *Townsend Letter* 6 (2014): 68-72.
[59] Dash, Sarah, Gerard Clarke, Michael Berk, and Felice N. Jacka. "The gut microbiome and diet in psychiatry: focus on depression." *Current opinion in psychiatry* 28, no. 1 (2015): 1-6.

THE NO-NONSENSE GUIDE TO DIGESTIVE DISEASES

[60] Groschwitz, Katherine R., and Simon P. Hogan. "Intestinal barrier function: molecular regulation and disease pathogenesis." *Journal of Allergy and Clinical Immunology* 124, no. 1 (2009): 3-20.

[61] Branum, Amy M., and Susan Lukacs. *Food allergy among US children: trends in prevalence and hospitalizations*. US Department of Health and Human Services, Centers for Disease Control and Prevention, National Center for Health Statistics, 2008.

[62] Gibson, Rosalind S. "The role of diet-and host-related factors in nutrient bioavailability and thus in nutrient-based dietary requirement estimates." Food and Nutrition Bulletin 28, no. 1_suppl1 (2007): S77-S100.

[63] Söderholm, Johan D., and Mary H. Perdue. "II. Stress and intestinal barrier function." *American Journal of Physiology-Gastrointestinal and Liver Physiology* 280, no. 1 (2001): G7-G13.

[64] Keszthelyi, Daniel, Gwen H. Dackus, Gwen M. Masclee, Joanna W. Kruimel, and Ad AM Masclee. "Increased proton pump inhibitor and NSAID exposure in irritable bowel syndrome: results from a case-control study." *BMC gastroenterology* 12, no. 1 (2012): 121.

HEALTHFUL PUBLICATIONS

[65] Purohit, Vishnudutt, J. Christian Bode, Christiane Bode, David A. Brenner, Mashkoor A. Choudhry, Frank Hamilton, Y. James Kang et al. "Alcohol, intestinal bacterial growth, intestinal permeability to endotoxin, and medical consequences: summary of a symposium." *Alcohol* 42, no. 5 (2008): 349-361.

[66] Bjarnason, I., P. Williams, P. Smethurst, T. J. Peters, and A. J. Levi. "Effect of non-steroidal anti-inflammatory drugs and prostaglandins on the permeability of the human small intestine." *Gut* 27, no. 11 (1986): 1292-1297.

[67] Myers, Stephen P. "The causes of intestinal dysbiosis: a review." *Altern Med Rev* 9, no. 2 (2004): 180-197.

[68] Teixeira, Tatiana FS, Maria Carmen Collado, Célia LLF Ferreira, Josefina Bressan, and G. Peluzio Maria do Carmo. "Potential mechanisms for the emerging link between obesity and increased intestinal permeability." *Nutrition research* 32, no. 9 (2012): 637-647.

[69] Sekirov, Inna, Shannon L. Russell, L. Caetano M. Antunes, and B. Brett Finlay. "Gut microbiota in health and disease." *Physiological reviews* 90, no. 3 (2010): 859-904.

[70] Factor, A. Possible Etiologic. "Increased Intestinal Permeability m Patients with Crohn's Disease and Their Relatives." *Annals of internal medicine* 105 (1986): 883-885.

[71] Fasano, Alessio, Tarcisio Not, Wenle Wang, Sergio Uzzau, Irene Berti, Alberto Tommasini, and Simeon E. Goldblum. "Zonulin, a newly discovered modulator of intestinal permeability, and its

expression in coeliac disease." *The Lancet* 355, no. 9214 (2000): 1518-1519.

[72] Spiller, R. C., D. Jenkins, J. P. Thornley, J. M. Hebden, T. Wright, M. Skinner, and K. R. Neal. "Increased rectal mucosal enteroendocrine cells, T lymphocytes, and increased gut permeability following acuteCampylobacter enteritis and in post-dysenteric irritable bowel syndrome." *Gut* 47, no. 6 (2000): 804-811.

[73] Troeger, Hanno, Christoph Loddenkemper, Thomas Schneider, Eckart Schreier, Hans-Joerg Epple, Martin Zeitz, Michael Fromm, and Joerg D. Schulzke. "Structural and functional changes of the duodenum in human norovirus infection." *Gut* 58, no. 8 (2009): 1070-1077.

[74] Kotanko, Peter, Mary Carter, and Nathan W. Levin. "Intestinal bacterial microflora—a potential source of chronic inflammation in patients with chronic kidney disease." *Nephrology Dialysis Transplantation* 21, no. 8 (2006): 2057-2060.

[75] Dalzell, A. M., N. S. Freestone, D. Billington, and D. P. Heaf. "Small intestinal permeability and orocaecal transit time in cystic fibrosis." *Archives of disease in childhood* 65, no. 6 (1990): 585-588.

[76] Bosi, E., L. Molteni, M. G. Radaelli, L. Folini, I. Fermo, E. Bazzigaluppi, L. Piemonti, M. R. Pastore, and R. Paroni. "Increased intestinal permeability precedes clinical onset of type 1 diabetes." *Diabetologia* 49, no. 12 (2006): 2824-

2827.

[77] Green, Peter HR, Kamran Rostami, and Michael N. Marsh. "Diagnosis of coeliac disease." *Best Practice & Research Clinical Gastroenterology* 19, no. 3 (2005): 389-400.

[78] Jackson, P. G., R. W. R. Baker, M. H. Lessof, Jean Ferrett, and D. M. MacDonald. "Intestinal permeability in patients with eczema and food allergy." *The Lancet* 317, no. 8233 (1981): 1285-1286.

[79] Matsuo, Hiroaki, Kenichi Morimoto, Tatsuya Akaki, Sakae Kaneko, K. Kusatake, T. Kuroda, H. Niihara, Michihiro Hide, and Eishin Morita. "Exercise and aspirin increase levels of circulating gliadin peptides in patients with wheat-dependent exercise-induced anaphylaxis." *Clinical & Experimental Allergy* 35, no. 4 (2005): 461-466.

[80] Hollander, Daniel. "Intestinal permeability, leaky gut, and intestinal disorders." *Current gastroenterology reports* 1, no. 5 (1999): 410-416.

[81] Bajaj, Jasmohan S., Jason M. Ridlon, Phillip B. Hylemon, Leroy R. Thacker, Douglas M. Heuman, Sean Smith, Masoumeh Sikaroodi, and Patrick M. Gillevet. "Linkage of gut microbiome with cognition in hepatic encephalopathy." *American Journal of Physiology-Gastrointestinal and Liver Physiology* 302, no. 1 (2012): G168-G175.

[82] Benard, Anne, Pierre Desreumeaux, Damien Huglo, Anne Hoorelbeke, André-Bernard Tonnel, and

THE NO-NONSENSE GUIDE TO DIGESTIVE DISEASES

Benoit Wallaert. "Increased intestinal permeability in bronchial asthma." *Journal of Allergy and Clinical Immunology* 97, no. 6 (1996): 1173-1178.

[83] Montalto, Massimo, Luca Santoro, Ferruccio D'Onofrio, Valentina Curigliano, Antonella Gallo, Dina Visca, Giovanni Cammarota, Antonio Gasbarrini, and Giovanni Gasbarrini. "Adverse reactions to food: allergies and intolerances." *Digestive Diseases* 26, no. 2 (2008): 96-103.

[84] Theoharides, Theoharis C., Robert Doyle, Konstantinos Francis, Pio Conti, and Dimitris Kalogeromitros. "Novel therapeutic targets for autism." *Trends in Pharmacological Sciences* 29, no. 8 (2008): 375-382.

[85] Brown, Christopher T., Austin G. Davis-Richardson, Adriana Giongo, Kelsey A. Gano, David B. Crabb, Nabanita Mukherjee, George Casella et al. "Gut microbiome metagenomics analysis suggests a functional model for the development of autoimmunity for type 1 diabetes." *PloS one* 6, no. 10 (2011): e25792.

[86] Holt, Erica M., Lyn M. Steffen, Antoinette Moran, Samar Basu, Julia Steinberger, Julie A. Ross, Ching-Ping Hong, and Alan R. Sinaiko. "Fruit and vegetable consumption and its relation to markers of inflammation and oxidative stress in adolescents." *Journal of the American Dietetic*

Association 109, no. 3 (2009): 414-421.
[87] Basu, Samar. "Radioimmunoassay of 15-keto-13, 14-dihydro-prostaglandin F2α: an index for inflammation via cyclooxygenase catalysed lipid peroxidation." *Prostaglandins, leukotrienes and essential fatty acids* 58, no. 5 (1998): 347-352.
[88] Spruss, Astrid, and Ina Bergheim. "Dietary fructose and intestinal barrier: potential risk factor in the pathogenesis of nonalcoholic fatty liver disease." *The Journal of nutritional biochemistry* 20, no. 9 (2009): 657-662.

[89] Melosky, Barb, Ron Burkes, Daniel Rayson, Thierry Alcindor, Neil Shear, and Mario Lacouture. "Management of skin rash during EGFR-targeted monoclonal antibody treatment for gastro intestinal malignancies: Canadian recommendations." *Current Oncology* 16, no. 1 (2009): 14-24.
[90] Rosenfeldt, Vibeke, Eva Benfeldt, Niels Henrik Valerius, Anders Pærregaard, and Kim Fleischer Michaelsen. "Effect of probiotics on gastrointestinal symptoms and small intestinal permeability in children with atopic dermatitis." *The Journal of pediatrics* 145, no. 5 (2004): 612-616.
[91] Solga, Steven F. "Probiotics can treat hepatic encephalopathy." *Medical hypotheses* 61, no. 2 (2003): 307-313.
[92] Buret, A. G., K. Mitchell, D. G. Muench, and K. G. E. Scott. "Giardia lamblia disrupts tight junctional ZO-1

and increases permeability in non-transformed human small intestinal epithelial monolayers: effects of epidermal growth factor." *Parasitology* 125, no. 01 (2002): 11-19.
[93] Surawicz, Christina M., Gary W. Elmer, Pieter Speelman, Lynne V. McFarland, Janet Chinn, and Gerald Van Belle. "Prevention of antibiotic-associated diarrhea by Saccharomyces boulardii: a prospective study." *Gastroenterology* 96, no. 4 (1989): 981-988.

[94] Isolauri, Erika, Heli Majamaa, Taina Arvola, Immo Rantala, Elina Virtanen, and Heikki Arvilommi. "Lactobacillus casei strain GG reverses increased intestinal permeability induced by cow milk in suckling rats." *Gastroenterology* 105, no. 6 (1993): 1643-1650.
[95] Wu, Guoyao, Yun-Zhong Fang, Sheng Yang, Joanne R. Lupton, and Nancy D. Turner. "Glutathione metabolism and its implications for health." *The Journal of nutrition* 134, no. 3 (2004): 489-492.
[96] Quigley, Eamonn MM. "Leaky gut–concept or clinical entity?." *Current opinion in gastroenterology* 32, no. 2 (2016): 74-79.
[97] Su, Liping, Le Shen, Daniel R. Clayburgh, Sam C. Nalle, Erika A. Sullivan, Jon B. Meddings, Clara Abraham, and Jerrold R. Turner. "Targeted epithelial

HEALTHFUL PUBLICATIONS

tight junction dysfunction causes immune activation and contributes to development of experimental colitis." *Gastroenterology* 136, no. 2 (2009): 551-563.
[98] Marchesi, Julian R., David H. Adams, Francesca Fava, Gerben DA Hermes, Gideon M. Hirschfield, Georgina Hold, Mohammed Nabil Quraishi et al. "The gut microbiota and host health: a new clinical frontier." *Gut* 65, no. 2 (2016): 330-339.
[99] Fukui, Hiroshi. "Endotoxin and other microbial translocation markers in the blood: A clue to understand leaky gut syndrome." *Cellular & Molecular Medicine: Open access* (2016).

[100] A Kohler, Cristiano, Michael Maes, Anastasiya Slyepchenko, Michael Berk, Marco Solmi, Krista L Lanctôt, and Andre F Carvalho. "The gut-brain axis, including the microbiome, leaky gut and bacterial translocation: mechanisms and pathophysiological role in Alzheimer's disease." *Current Pharmaceutical Design* 22, no. 40 (2016): 6152-6166.
[101] Sherwin, Eoin, Kieran Rea, Timothy G. Dinan, and John F. Cryan. "A gut (microbiome) feeling about the brain." *Current opinion in gastroenterology* 32, no. 2 (2016): 96-102.
[102] Kato, Takayuki, Yasushi Honda, Yusuke Kurita, Akito Iwasaki, Takamitsu Sato, Takaomi Kessoku, Shiori Uchiyama et al. "Lubiprostone improves intestinal permeability in humans, a novel therapy

for the leaky gut: A prospective randomized pilot study in healthy volunteers." *PloS one* 12, no. 4 (2017): e0175626.

[103] Kwak, Dong Shin, Oh Young Lee, Kang Nyeong Lee, Dae Won Jun, Hang Lak Lee, Byung Chul Yoon, and Ho Soon Choi. "The Effect of DA-6034 on Intestinal Permeability in an Indomethacin-Induced Small Intestinal Injury Model." *Gut and liver* 10, no. 3 (2016): 406.

Printed in Great Britain
by Amazon